KEEPING IT REAL
with
ARTHRITIS

IMAGINEWE
Publishers

ImagineWe Publishers
A Global Publisher

IMAGINEWE
Publishers™

This book is an original publication of ImagineWe Publishers.

Published by: ImagineWe, LLC
ImagineWe Publishers
247 Market Street, Suite 201
Lockport, NY 14094
United States
www.imaginewepublishers.com

© 2022 ImagineWe, LLC

Edited by: Samantha Moss
Illustrations and Book Cover Designed by: Loren Mendoza
Book Project Idea by: Effie Koliopoulos

www.keepingitrealwitharthritisbook.com

ISBN: 978-1-946512-71-0 (Paperback)
ISBN: 978-1-946512-72-7 (Hardcover)
Library of Congress Control Number: 2022919933

First Edition: December 2022

PRINTED IN THE UNITED STATES OF AMERICA

We are always looking for new authors. For more information, please visit the website listed above.
To shop our selection of books and merchandise you can visit: www.shop.imaginewepublishers.com

To all those who made this book possible,
thank you for shining your light and making this world a better place.

Special Thanks to

The HealtheVoices Impact Fund that helped bring this project to life. This is a grant program that supports innovative efforts by health advocates to serve and assist patient communities. The Fund was established at the Community Foundation of New Jersey and awards projects that align with the Janssen charitable giving mission, to advance healing for patients.

Learn more about the grant here:
www.healthevoices.com

Contributing Authors

Contents

INTRODUCTION

I must admit, writing this introduction was probably one of the hardest parts of putting this book together. Thinking of what to say was a little overwhelming. After all, the people featured in the book are quite simply put- my heroes. As you read through the stories, you may very well come to find that they are yours too.

As I released any anxiety surrounding this project, I reminded myself of the purpose, the reason, the cause, or the why; whatever you want to call it. But before sharing that, I want to discuss a part of my arthritis journey that played a pivotal role in the making of this book.

When I was diagnosed with juvenile arthritis eighteen years ago in 2004, social media wasn't quite on the scene yet. Popular social outlets in the early 2000s ceased to exist, as new innovative ideas that we see today took shape. But I started to wonder. What if the social media platforms we have become accustomed to over the last couple of decades are no longer available to us? While that is unlikely to happen, we never know. Nevertheless, it made me think of creating something more tangible and long-lasting for people of today and future generations to come. Well, you may be asking why?

Despite a few online blogs, forums, message boards, pamphlets, or magazines at a medical provider office, that only featured people of a certain demographic and age, resources and support were sparse back in the day when I was diagnosed. Imagine for a moment this is all you had to rely on today. Maybe you don't have to imagine because you lived it. Of course, some generations ago people had no internet and barely any treatment options. It is my hope that this book will show us just how far we have come, but how much further we still need to go in providing ample resources, awareness, education, and overall support.

Now fast forward to the present moment. We have so many places to turn to for respite, connection, and resources. The worldwide web and various social platforms have allowed me the privilege to meet people from all over the world who are living with arthritis and their supporters. I know now how extremely isolating, lonely, and scary it can be not to know anyone your age, in your city, state, country, or ethnic background with arthritis.

Reading other people's stories is what I like to call 'real-life education.' It forces us to become open-minded and view our experiences through the lens of another. My other three hopes with this book are for supporters to have their voices heard too, for people in society to have more compassion and empathy towards those of us dealing with this disease, and for awareness that people are more than a diagnosis. Those with lived experience and clinical experience are both experts. It's crucial to listen to all sides to make substantial movement forward within patient care, medical care, and research.

Going back to social media, you will notice in this book, there is no section for resources or any mention of social media accounts from those who submitted a story. The stories featured are the resource. I came to this conclusion organically as I looked back at how it all started. In 2017, I started to feature interviews with people in the arthritis community on my blog Rising Above rheumatoid arthritis. It was far from a viral sensation, but that didn't matter nor was it why I wanted to do it.

Connecting with like-minded people was a special, refreshing, and invigorating experience in and of itself because it helped me heal emotionally from a complex total knee replacement surgery. It was an exciting time because I felt a surge of courage to branch out into the world of advocacy full-on.

This small step eventually evolved into featuring more stories from people who lived all over the world on my other social platforms. This showed me even more that arthritis didn't care who you were or most importantly, where you lived. The illustrated world map you will find in this book, following this introduction, is telling and can spark interesting debates. Do certain areas of the world see more arthritis or chronic illness cases than others? Do people not want to talk about it as openly as other parts of the world? Do some areas have more or less access to medical care, resources, and support? While not every part of the world is represented here, hopefully, one day it will be.

One common thread through most of the stories I began to hear, as I started my advocacy work, was the fact that arthritis doesn't only affect someone on a physical level. I knew this to be true from my own lived experience. That is why I decided to make themes a central focus of this book. Where people could share stories about life with arthritis on all levels from physical health, mental health, social lives, relationships, faith and spirituality, finances, and work and career life balance.

For those of you who made this book possible by sharing your story, I can't thank you enough. Your real-life experiences, thoughts, and perspectives, are valuable resources. Each of you is helping to pave the way for others by shining a light on both your triumphs and difficulties. But most importantly holding space for people to be heard, seen, and validated. It's not always easy to be vulnerable and open.

Sometimes it can be exhausting and not something you want to do. Other times it can be deeply fulfilling as it allows you to connect with people who share similar, if not the same, experiences as you. Holding space for those not ready to share, or who don't want to at all, is also important. Most of all, giving grace to ourselves throughout our arthritis journey is crucial. The same goes for those in our lives

"Each of you is helping to pave the way for others by shining a light on both your triumphs and difficulties. But most importantly holding space for people to be heard, seen, and validated."

who support us and are trying their best. These stories are bringing awareness to our own everyday realities, making us feel less alone. They also bring awareness to the world about misconceptions, stigmas, and unmet needs through your experiences.

To those who read this book, thank you for giving it a chance. I can mention what I would want you to take away from it after reading it, but that is not my place. It will be personal for everyone. But I hope you can pass on the wisdom from these stories and share it with those you do know.

There is no doubt that the arthritis community has an unmatched sense of comradery. I hope you take a moment to be proud of yourself for being part of something bigger and creating change that is much needed in our community.

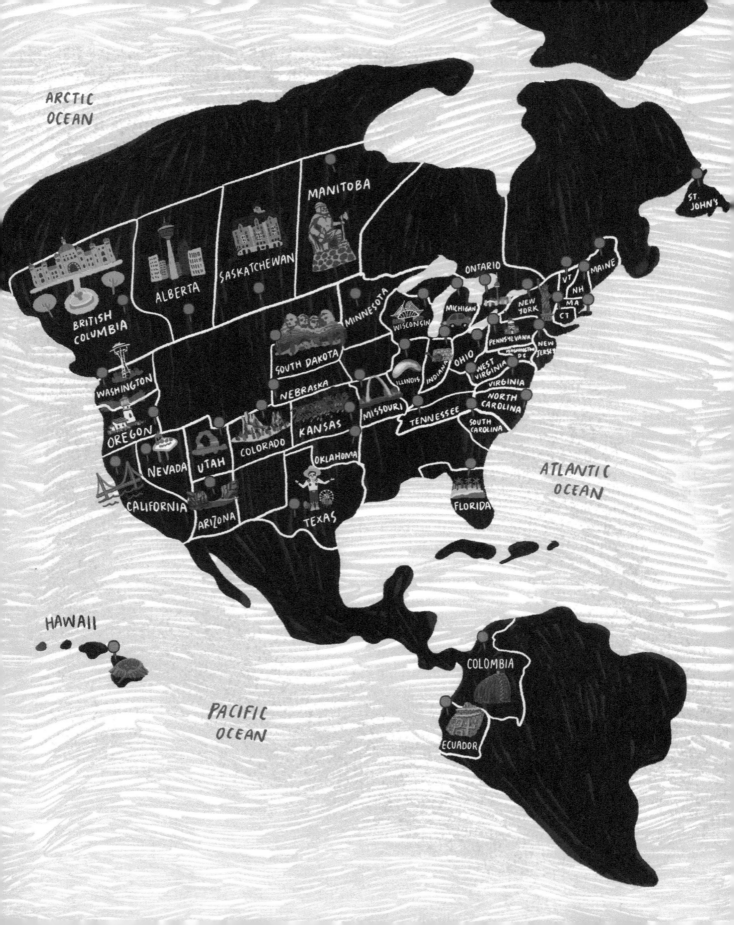

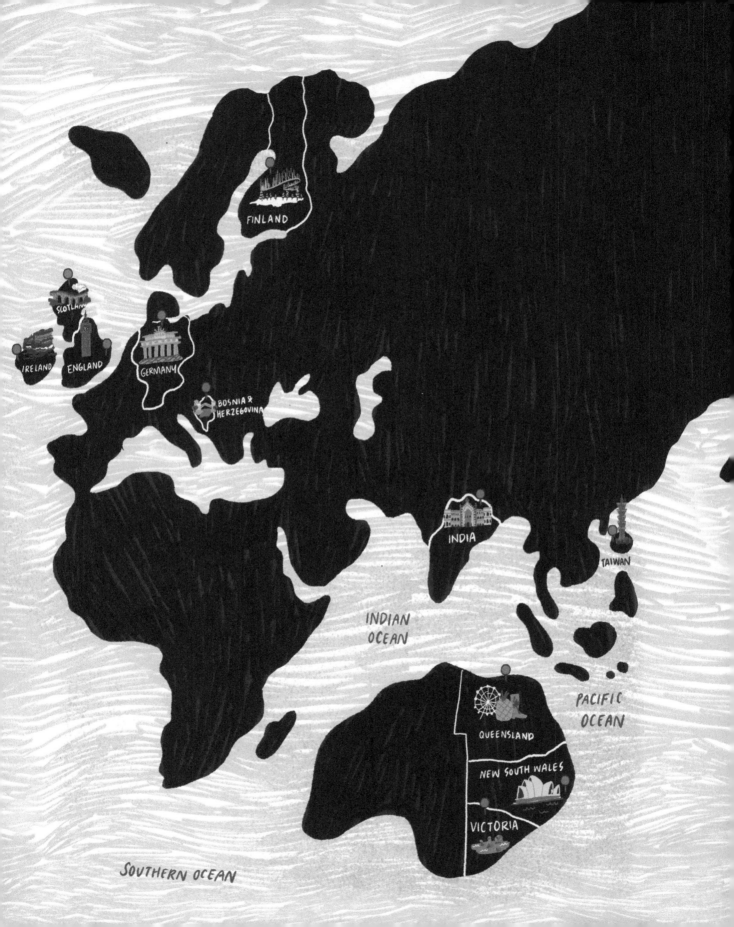

FINLAND

SCOTLAND

IRELAND

ENGLAND

GERMANY

BOSNIA & HERZEGOVINA

INDIA

TAIWAN

INDIAN OCEAN

PACIFIC OCEAN

QUEENSLAND

NEW SOUTH WALES

VICTORIA

SOUTHERN OCEAN

ARTHRITIS SUPPORTER

Stories

Steven Moustos

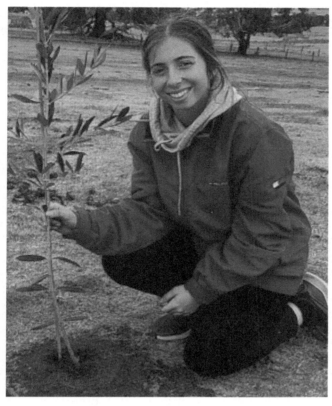

"Have hope your child will get better."

Father Versus Arthritis

I could write a book with many chapters relating to my clinical research into juvenile rheumatoid arthritis. Instead I am going to write a chapter about myself, a father of a daughter who was diagnosed with JRA 18 years ago. To most people, my story will sound strange because, "kids do not get arthritis as this is an elderly disease." But for families who have experienced this disease, my story will be identical to theirs.

Growing Pains

Most people believe when a child complains about sore joints, it's because they are going through a growth spurt. This may be true in some cases, or it could be recovering from athletics and sporting injuries. But for a small population of kids,

it's the effects of JRA. When I became aware there was a problem with my daughter's mobility and attended the local general practitioner for advice, he said, "kids do not get arthritis." Friends, family, and grandparents would say the same thing. To be fair, I too was ignorant and uneducated back then about this disease. It's the last thing a parent would expect, that their child has an arthritic condition. I attended many kids birthday parties where my daughter was invited, and we would go to the park and playgrounds often. It was here I gradually noticed my daughter's reduced mobility compared to other kids of similar age.

The Diagnosis

Not only did my daughter's mobility get worse, but she also developed a hard lump on her wrist. I suspected this may be the cause of her mobility problems, but then she could not even go up the stairs to her bedroom, hold her arm high enough to brush her own hair, or clean herself up after going to the toilet.

We were referred to see a surgeon regarding the growing lump on my daughter's wrist. The surgeon arranged for blood tests and requested an MRI to confirm what this growth was. We met the surgeon after all these tests were performed and he suspected JRA. He was not an expert for this disease, so we were referred to a pediatric rheumatoid specialist. The specialist confirmed JRA based on elevated pathology markers, as well as topical swelling around her joints and the MRI diagnosis. I was no longer ignorant that this was an elderly disease.

How Bad Can It Get

My daughter was diagnosed at age six. By age seven this disease had not only affected all her joints, it had spread to her neck and jaw. There were also concerns it had spread to the eye muscles. Worse still was my daughter would often get hives and skin rashes, all made worse when she had an adverse reaction to prescription anti-inflammatory medication. We would attend physiotherapy and occupational therapy on a monthly basis which started to instill the seriousness of this disease and how it was progressing.

My daughter could not take any medication and was at the mercy of JRA which was relentless and unforgiving at this time. She would get sore after eating foods, so much of it was mashed to minimize chewing. Her neck could not move from side to side any further than 15 degrees and attempting to do so caused migraines. If you imagine what tunnel vision would be like, this was tunnel-torso. Further reality set in when we kept her stroller, using it to take her to primary school, to minimize walking and reduce the pain. She is not one to complain, yet I would notice the tear in the corner of her eye as she held her hand and wrist inside her clothing, to find a posture which minimized pain.

The Cross Road

Her specialist may as well have told me my daughter had cancer with all the emotions that go with such a diagnosis. There were new generation drugs and biological agents that were being developed back in the mid 2000's, aimed at suppressing the auto-immune disorders that occur with this disease. Before this, a child would take half or a quarter of an anti-inflammatory tablet, because a full tablet was an adult dosage and kids weigh less. This was the extent of any active research into this disease at the time. Unfortunately, JRA affects a small population of kids, so no drug company is going to invest in a cure. Not only was I feeling helpless, but there was also no foreseeable help. By this stage my daughters ESR pathology result was 56 when it should be less than three for this age group. In addition, having elevated white cell count and CRP levels were all indicative of her own body's immune system believing her joints were an infection, and therefore attacking them as though they were a foreign object.

I did not agree to these new generation medications which became the go-to-drugs. In fairness they are designed to slow down JRA and joint damage, but these are not a cure. I took a big risk on behalf of my daughter who could have ended up with serious, permanent long term joint damage that was irreversible. Instead, I had another idea and different treatment plan which has become the backbone of my personal clinical research into JRA. I will not go into any further details as this chapter is about my experience.

I Know What It Is Like

I was actively involved with the Arthritis Foundation in Victoria Australia, where we would attend camps and family group outings all intended to provide a support network for parents and JRA kids. We participated for several years even after my daughter's remission. I found some resentment from parents after they saw my daughter's mobility improve, as well as becoming aware of her remission. I no longer felt I belonged to this group and chose to no longer participate.

I understand what families go through because I have been there too. I know what it's like to carry a child upstairs because their knees hurt and to piggy-back a child to school to "save the knees" for some sports related activities. I know how to neglect my other kids because one is unwell and needs all my attention. I know what it's like to worry about a child having yet another theater session for cortisone. I know what it's like to have financial difficulties because you have to take time off work for many appointments and the cost of treatment. I know what it's like to watch my child take many tablets first thing in the morning. I know how frustrating it is to search for answers and find little about what causes this disease and how to cure it. I know what it's like to go to a public playground and watch other kids run around whilst my child is keeping still because they are in pain. I know what it's like dealing with some medical officers who have limited understanding of this disease. I know what it's like to spend countless hours researching and web browsing to look for answers, treatment options and cures. And you too, know what it is like.

Have Hope

By age nine, my daughter was in complete remission. I still remember the medical specialist appointment where she would yet again be lying on a procedural bed, having the specialist topically feel for swelling around her joints. On this occasion it was different. There was no swelling to be found. Leading up to this my daughter was becoming more mobile, even riding a push bike. As a precaution her specialist asked for blood tests to review JRA markers. Results came back normal, showing no JRA. Blood tests were taken again two weeks later, as the specialist had suggested an error or mix up may have occurred in the pathology laboratory. He had never seen remission this fast or in this young. Following tests again confirmed no active JRA.

At age 10 my daughter joined a soccer club where she played until 12. She picked up this sport again when she turned 18 and played striker for her university's soccer team. From age 9 to 12 she rode dirt bikes competing in a junior class. Overlapping all this, she participated in horse riding, jumping and dressage for some 10 years. All these activities need strong knees and are impossible with active JRA.

She is now 24 and has successfully completed all physical requirements to join the Australian Navy. The armed forces physical entrance requirements are demanding and any hint of any permanent or long-term joint damage from JRA will ensure you do not get accepted.

Looking For A Cure

As difficult as this was for me, I can say much good has come out of it. I was inspired and encouraged to find a cure for this disease. If it was not for my daughter's disease, I would not have looked for a cure or invested 18 years of clinical research to understand this disease.

Laura Kelly

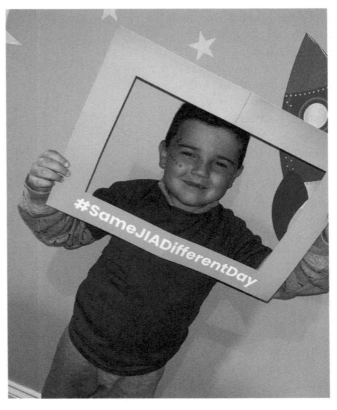

"JIA warriors!"

My six year old son was diagnosed with enthesitis related arthritis in January 2022. As a caregiver this was such an emotional and stressful time. Many days have been filled with tears but we have to put a brave face on. Nothing prepares you for the surgery, drugs, pain and side effects you will face. How do we cope when our world essentially comes crashing down? The last thing you want for your child is to face any difficulties in their life.

Our experience so far is very much still ongoing. Trying to find the right treatment that works for our boy is proving not as easy as we thought. Anyone who is caring for someone with juvenile idiopathic arthritis, hang in there, look for the positives in any situation. I pray my son continues to fight this every single day. Some days he asks, *"why me? Why do I have arthritis? I want to be normal."*

I wish I had all the answers. Even at such a young age it has a negative effect on his mental health which is so worrying. But we are not alone. Facebook groups have been a godsend and it is a comfort to know so many people are going through the same thing. JIA is not widely spoken about enough. I personally had no idea it was even a thing before my son was diagnosed. Those horrible first few months going from carrying him around unable to walk, the first general anesthetic, to now steroid weekly injections, monthly blood tests and new flares coming all the time! The side effects, headaches, not being able to sleep, the tiredness, can all truly eat you up.

This book will be an opening for everyone to speak about JIA and RA. Every single person fighting this, you are warriors and I take my hat off to each and every one of you. I hope our journey will end very soon but if not, we keep going and fighting.

Erin Rounds

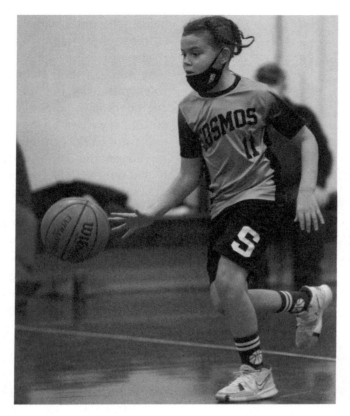

"It's OK. You've got this. Breathe."

Where There's A Will There's A Way
Will Aviles, age 10 as told by mom Erin Rounds

The early morning light was dim. Outside Will's window birds chirped and twittered, but he couldn't hear them through his tears.

"*Moooom*!" he cried.

Like she had every morning for weeks, Will's mom rushed in to comfort him and carry his inflamed body to the bathroom to pee and sit in a hot shower.

"*It's OK. You've got this. Breathe.*"

At breakfast she mixed turmeric powder into his OJ, and gave him another dose of motrin. At the end of the day the school bus had to wait for him to make it down the hallway and by the time he got to her building, she had to meet him in the lobby and piggyback him up the stairs.

"*It's OK. You've got this. Breathe.*"

The insurance had finally approved a switch in biologics, so she prayed these days would soon be behind him.

Two weeks later Will sat in pediatric oncology for a three hour infusion of his new medicine. The nurses were doting, there were snacks and a tablet. But the best part was when the drips were done. Will ran down the hallway yelling, "I feel great!"

Seven months later, after a successful soccer season, Will's mom sat in the stands of a basketball game. The scoreboard clock ticked down, and Will glanced up as he dribbled. There was his mom cheering the loudest.

"*You've got this, Will!*"

He inhaled deeply and pushed through the pain.

"*I've got this.*"

Yvonne Codd

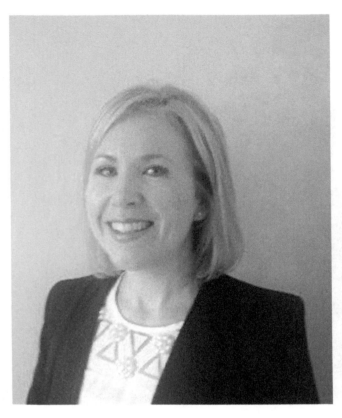

"Arthritis affects your whole life – not just your joints!"

An Occupational Therapy Perspective to Inflammatory Arthritis Management

The importance of early access to medical and drug therapy management, to support best outcomes in the management of inflammatory arthritis, is well recognized. The advancements in drug therapy to decrease disease activity and improve rates of remission has been a welcome addition in the field of rheumatology. However, despite these positives, many people with inflammatory arthritis continue to experience disease symptoms which interrupt their function and their ability to engage in previously enjoyed life roles, such as employment, parenting, and social roles.

At its core, occupational therapy is a healthcare profession which has a broader perspective on health. It looks wider than disease management to treat the visible and invisible impacts of an illness, or injury on a person's function and how they manage their home, work, leisure and social roles and tasks. occupational therapists work with each person to help them to manage their impacts, so that they can enjoy the things they need to do and want to do in their own everyday life.

Given the age profile of this client group, a new diagnosis often occurs at a time when people are settling down into adult life properly and thinking about career and family life. Often the primary focus in early arthritis management is to identify the optimum medication and dosage to manage the disease. However, life does not stop during the disease stabilization phase, and therefore, active monitoring and support with life role engagement is also important. Research on employment and arthritis reports that the vast majority of those who leave work due to their arthritis do not return [1]. Therefore, concurrent work supports during disease stabilization to support work role retention is key.

While it was hoped that the newer rheumatology medications would naturally improve life role retention, this has not borne out in the literature as may have been expected. Work loss among employees with inflammatory arthritis remains a challenge [2-5]. Similarly, engagement in parenting [6] and social roles [7] is increasingly recognized as compromised.

Occupational therapy interventions focus on how current roles are impacted because of the diagnosis, plus the development of strategies to support people to continue to retain and enjoy those roles as they go on through their life course. Understanding and managing the visible and invisible symptoms and how they are impacting on function is key to supporting people to retain role engagement in work, parenting relationships and social roles.

Visible symptoms can include swelling, stiffness, heat, loss of strength or movement. Invisible symptoms are just that – invisible, every bit as real, and can include pain, fatigue, stress, anxiety or worry, guilt, self-expectation, and expectation of others. Interventions that manage these impacts well are the ones which consider the:

- Person at the center and their own experience of their visible and invisible symptoms;
- Person in their role (work, parent, etc) looking at the physical and social environment, the physical demands and the emotional demands, the routines and patterns that accompany this role;
- Outside of the role factors such as the commute, commitments, and responsibilities (family and financial), supports, routines and patterns of conscious self-care, sleep architecture and joy.

Life roles like work or parenting can be challenging, because of the physical restrictions and also the emotional restrictions associated with disease, which can result in altered capacity for the role. A change of capacity physically, and/or emotionally for a role, can shift the dynamics in relationships, add to guilt and a sense of burden and require some delegation of tasks associated with those roles. There is a complexity to asking for help and how it relates to control, grieving, ableism, and independence which must be acknowledged. Delegation of previously held roles and responsibilities is very personal. For some it is a relief to have the challenge recognized and supported and allows a freedom to redirect energies to other tasks. However, many people with arthritis experience hurt, upset, and guilt at the delegation of 'their' jobs, and an additional burden and pressure to manage.

An individualized approach is necessary to ensure the right type of support for each person. Identity is intrinsically linked with roles and for many, particularly those in the early stage of their diagnosis, their paid occupation or parenting role defines them. Therefore difficulty with role engagement, or role performance, can add additional worry, guilt, and hurt [2-6]. Help and support from others can be helpful, but only if it is wanted. Perceived 'forced help', or perceived 'forced delegation' of tasks, can have additional emotional consequences and add to burden. Conversely, it is important to acknowledge that it's okay to need help and we all need help at times. It is part of life so be kind to yourself in the process. Sometimes help affords a breathing space and that is valuable too. Awareness of the complexities of help is important, both for those who live with arthritis and for all of their supporters.

In addition to the healthcare supports available to support life role engagement, there are many charity groups in my country (Arthritis Ireland, in Ireland), work support grants (workplace equipment adaptation grant, employee retention grant, wage subsidy grant), re-training services (Springboard, county partnerships, local library services, education and training Boards), local community groups (mother and toddler Groups, Men's Shed), as well as online groups (Arthritis Ireland, Rheum to THRIVE) which can provide support.

Early intervention is proven to support best outcomes, whereas delayed access to therapy usually requires more complex stepped-care interventions, with greater challenges to achieve good outcomes. However, timing for services can be complex and readiness for help is key. Therefore, a flexible 'right advice' and the 'right time' approach may be more impactful. Regardless, it is important to know that addressing life roles is within the scope of rheumatology clinical practice and therefore it might be helpful to discuss any work, parenting, driving concerns, etc with your healthcare provider and ask to see the occupational therapist!

Latika Gupta

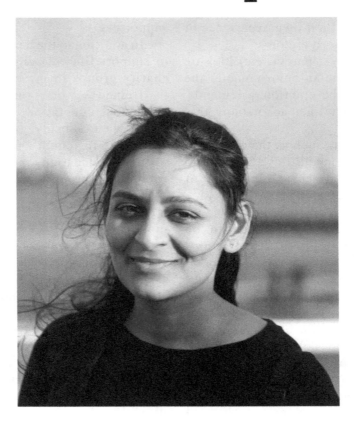

"When you see the same patients again and again, there's a relationship and a bond that you develop."

A lady (Mrs. DS) in her 30's, living in India, had antisynthetase syndrome (ASSD) and associated interstitial lung disease (ILD). It took a while to diagnose, as ILD was insidious to start with, and muscle involvement occurred much later.

When first seen in the rheumatology outpatient clinic of a tertiary care hospital in Northern India, she was commenced on high-dose steroids and azathioprine, and soon started showing signs of improvement. Unfortunately, the responses did not last too long, as she had an episode of dengue infection and was admitted to the hospital. In fact, she was in and out of the hospital a few times, with different complications from treatments, like a urine infection. So, we had to discontinue azathioprine and try other treatments. Unfortunately, her disease relentlessly flared every time the steroid dose was reduced, suggesting no drug was working for her.

Despite her misery, she had such a bright and warm personality. She was a teacher, and I was impressed by her zeal to educate and empower kids. Meeting her would make anyone's day, as she had prominent undaunted optimism and the spirit to brave all odds that were somewhat unique. At the same time, it was heartbreaking to see her, gradually and silently, struggling to continue working at school and perform adequately at her job. Eventually, as lung function declined, she had to request to be moved to a classroom on ground level, as she couldn't climb stairs anymore. Processing paperwork to secure funding and permissions for advanced treatments was yet another silent sign of a failure to treat her condition well. Then there were the social issues. She was the breadwinner of the family, and that put her in a tight spot in keeping the household going.

There were also cultural complexities; women in India struggle to exercise free will, and avail the opportunity to take independent decisions regarding their own health. Every time we decided on a new immunosuppressant, we went over all the potential adverse events, effects, and pros and cons. It was always a challenge due to conflicting family opinions. Then there were financial issues, as insurance cover could not be availed.

She couldn't work any more when she had relapsed for the third time. However, she was still very positive, and she told me she was turning entrepreneurial, and hoping to work from home soon by establishing a coaching center for school children. By this time, she also felt motivated to spread awareness about ASSD. She had read all about the condition, and learned how difficult antisynthetase is to diagnose, so she joined several support groups and felt committed to spreading awareness. She discussed the inception of the Myositis India patient support group, to educate and empower Indian patients with myositis.

Meanwhile, to tackle her disease, we arrived at the very difficult decision to use the Rituxan injection. It required hospital admissions, and adequate funding. While we got around to doing that she developed an extremely rare complication, reported only aneEEotally with Rituxan, called ARDS (acute respiratory syndrome). It's a condition where fluid in the lungs limits normal breathing and oxygenation, often requiring ventilatory support. Sadly, she deteriorated within hours of getting Rituxan.

She was admitted to the intensive care unit and, after a nine-day long battle, we lost her to the condition. She also left behind a young grieving daughter who was in primary school. It was a difficult day for me as a doctor. On January 1st, she and her daughter visited me with a thank you card, for finding a way to save her mother's life and deciding on a new medicine that would hopefully bring some relief. I could not bear the thought that just a week later her mother was battling for her life in the ICU, and eventually succumbed to the condition.

It was heartbreaking to lose her, and really led me to rethink managing chronic conditions. When a doctor meets the same patient, again and again, a strong bond develops over time. There's a technical aspect of expertise and opinion as a doctor and a human connection that goes way beyond. The responsibilities of being a doctor include being objective, responsible, meticulous, and logical at all junctures, and providing information with the patient's right to autonomy and justice. Despite human emotions, bonds, and connections, steering clear of countertransference is advisable, though also considered inevitable by some. For carers of patients with chronic diseases, this shall remain an ongoing debate.

Mrs. DS did leave us, but her spirit does live on. She couldn't take Myositis India forward but hopefully one day another special one will lead the group with her vision and mission.

MENTAL

HEALTH

Stories

Tina Jovanovska

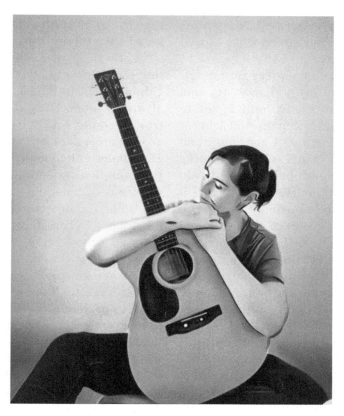

""There's no easy way out, there's no shortcut home" and as hard as it is to push through, in the end any success is better than having none at all."

What is life with rheumatoid arthritis? Honestly it's the easiest yet hardest question to answer. If you had asked me this question a few years back I would have gone into detail about every painful experience I had endured to date. Ask me now and my response will be that my body is at war with itself and I have the battle scars to prove it.

Along with this illness I have been diagnosed with two other autoimmune diseases and the joy of additional complications these conditions bring. Since diagnosis I have had multiple surgeries and currently take nine different medications a day and a bi-monthly infusion, along with multiple specialist reviews and general care. My 97 year old grandmother and I compete as to who has the most pills to pop in a day and right now we are tied.

Like many of us here, I had to teach my body to adjust, and yet six years later my head still goes in the toilet bowl from time to time, rejecting all the toxic chemicals. There, right there, is one thing that scares me. To be able to live a "healthy, normal life" we go to an oncology clinic to see the nurses put on gowns from head to toe to be covered because they are handling a toxic substance. We sit there in the chair and watch them inject that toxic substance into our bodies. Conflicting thoughts cross my mind on how I can live with this poison in me, and yet without it I struggle to live at all.

From the day I was diagnosed my specialist painted a picture of my future. He told me straight out that I would have to have several surgeries that will leave me with minimal mobility. I had heard this over and over again, and when the time came to do the surgeries I was fine with it as it was drilled into me, but emotionally I still struggled to acknowledge and accept what was happening. My most recent experience has stolen what I loved doing the most, playing music.

This year I had my second surgery on my left wrist, now when I pick up my guitar to try and play I am lucky to last a whole minute before bursting out into tears from the pain and lack of function from my hand. I hate it! I get angry and confused and only know that this is the beginning of saying goodbye to something I love. How do you argue with this condition? How do you tell it that it's stolen something so important to you? You don't. I have learned with patience, training and alternate means, it is possible to get back what has been taken from you. But the thing is, you need to want to fight for it. In the words of Robert Tepper "there's no easy way out, there's no shortcut home" and as hard as it is to push through, in the end any success is better than having none at all.

I never understood why people would call this condition an "invisible illness until an experience in a shopping center. When you see me, I appear to be a young, healthy woman, but I hold a disability parking pass. Now, even though I have every right to park in a disabled car spot, I choose to only do so on days I really need it. There was a time I was having a bad flare day and happened to be in the car with my close friend. We decided to park in a disabled car spot. A lady stood at the center's doors staring at my friend and I coming out of the car. She was shaking her head at us and giving a facial expression of death stares. My friend, being protective, had every motion of anger and wanted to walk up to her and confront her about what she doesn't know. I pulled her back and said it's fine and to let it be.

A few months later I had surgery on my knee. We had parked in a disabled car spot again and before we even got out of the vehicle a bystander stood there watching us with glary eyes. As they saw my friend come around and assist me with the crutches, in a matter of a few seconds that bystander provided a genuine sympathetic smile, simply because they saw a mobility device.

That day I learned and saw first hand the meaning of "invisible illness" and yes, I do have a regret of not letting my friend correct the first lady. People judge, it is natural but how do you teach them not to if you don't say anything. Today if this was to happen, I would honestly be more than happy to undress myself so they can see every scar I have on my body from all the surgeries.

Let's drop in Covid. When it first came out into the world my reaction didn't change. Because I didn't need to adjust what I had been doing for all these years. Hand sanitizing and staying away from people with viruses, when everyone else around me was in a panic and trying to be cautious. Surprisingly, I thought to myself I was in a good position, this was nothing new for me, this is how it's always been.

Being immunocompromised has already taught me how to protect myself as much as possible from viruses. Generally catching a cold or flu was dangerous for me and like clockwork, without fail, I'd always be taken to hospital for treatment for pneumonia. But like everyone, no matter how much I did to protect myself, in the end I did get Covid to a severe extent. Yes it was horrible and I had to take special medication to treat it and it took me what felt like a lifetime for it to pass. But that's just it, it passed it and as the world slowly settles back to its old self and routines, again nothing changes for me. Having this condition I still need to carry out every day with caution.

So how do we carry ourselves through this crazy life? I fall into the fortunate category with this illness. I have been lucky enough from day one to have the right medical support and relationships with family and friends that got me through the tough times, but yet the struggle is still there.

The one thing that has been here with me from the core is music. Day in and day out I will put those earphones in and blast the tunes of songs that will get me through, keep me going and soldier on.

There are thousands of words I could write here on what the challenges have been on this journey, and yet these are the ones that standout the most.

This isn't much but I would like to acknowledge and dedicate this short story to every medical specialist, nurse, healthcare provider, my family, best friend, friends and employers, that have all been part of my life and stood by me while learning how to live life with RA.

Carrie Kellenberger

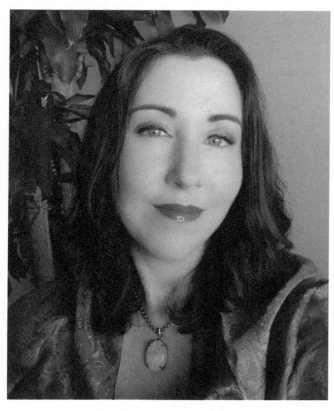

"When life decided to take me on a journey with chronic illness, I went with it just like I went with all the adventures I've had with travel. Although I've had to give up things I love the most, I found other things that I love equally as much. In the midst of illness, I could still choose how I wanted to live each day within my limits and who I wanted to be. I used to be a traveler, but now my days are filled with helping others navigate their own journeys. And we can take those journeys together. After all, the point is to keep moving forward."

"Y*ou're going to do what?*," my mother asked as we were driving home from our family cottage in Canada in July 2002.

"I'm moving abroad for a year to teach English and then I'm going to travel and see the world.," I replied.

The look on her face! *"No, you are not! Why on earth would you want to do that, Carrie? It's not safe."*

In 2002, I was 26 years old and I was longing for different experiences before settling down into the life that was expected of me. But like always, life takes you down a different path. And my life took me to China and countless other countries since.

Now, if anyone had ever told me I'd move abroad and not come home. I never would've believed them. At that time, I had no idea that I would live in China for three years. I just knew I was getting my teaching certificate, and I'd be halfway across the world by that time next summer.

The health problems that had plagued me since childhood seemed under control when I made the decision to move abroad. The low back pain and joint pain was gone. I was in good shape. I felt fit and ready. After all, what could happen in a year? A lot, as it turns out, but I will get to that part of my story soon.

Shortly after arriving in China in early 2003, I learned there was a mysterious virus called SARS going around. Travelers were being called back to their home countries. Before I could even consider booking a flight, SARS had already popped up in Toronto, so I decided to stay put.

It didn't take long. By summer 2003, we were in the full swing of things with classes. My boss and I also began prepping for a big talent show for foreigners in Changchun, China at the end of the year. (That's how my music and television career started in Asia.) After participating in that show, we flew to Beijing to participate in a two-week reality tv show for foreign performers from all over China that aired during Lunar New Year in 2004.

I really learned how to roll with things during my first year in China. What a valuable lesson this was! Learning how to adapt to changes came from traveling and life abroad where life isn't anything like what we're used to back home.

These lessons helped me for what was to come.

It was shortly after the television show that those pesky back, shoulder, and neck problems returned. Then it started affecting my legs and joints. There were days I'd wake up and I couldn't move my head, lift my arm, or put weight on my left foot. My knees would swell up and down regularly.

I had severe morning stiffness and unrelenting chronic pain, but it was easy to brush it off because of my lifestyle. I also had crushing fatigue, but by that time I'd met a man and fell in love and we found ourselves in Taipei, Taiwan in early 2006. And we took every opportunity that came our way.

In retrospect, I was doing too much and burning the candle at both ends, but isn't that what we're supposed to do in our 20s? We're supposed to be having fun and experiencing life! Grab those reins. Seize the day! Do it all and do it with no regrets.

And so I did, and I pushed the discomfort and pain to the side and convinced myself that what I was experiencing was normal. And because I had been normalizing that pain since my teens through a lot of athletics and I was able to push through it, it was easy to convince myself that everyone felt that way.

Two years went by in Taipei with the same symptoms, but I kept on going and saying yes to everything, until I couldn't.

In February 2009, I woke up to a heavy feeling in my legs. It felt like my legs, hips and lower back were filling up with cement. The next day, I woke up with hot, red swollen knees and my feet were starting to swell. Every time I stood up, it felt like my legs were going to snap. ER attention was needed.

Even sitting in the wheelchair was painful. I kept trying to get up to alleviate this horrendous pain, and of course, my legs wouldn't support me.

The ER doc took one look at me and asked me if I had been tested for rheumatoid arthritis. He aspirated my knees, did some tests, and sent me home with anti-inflammatories. But the swelling came back and I was still in a wheelchair when we returned a week later. He thought I had something called ankylosing spondylitis. They didn't have an AS specialist on staff, so he referred me to another hospital where my AS diagnosis was confirmed within a week.

Sure enough, the diagnosis was correct and that was my answer to 15 years of chronic pain. We now know I have axial spondyloarthritis and psoriatic arthritis. I started treatment and eventually the inflammation went down. Things were improving. I was back at the gym, back on stage, and we went full tilt with our travels. But then July 2014 rolled around and the swelling was back. I was out of remission from inflammatory arthritis.

It's 2022 and I'm still living in Asia. I've been here for 18 years. I own my own business and assist teachers in finding teaching positions for their adventures abroad in Asia. I'm also a health advocate for foreigners, in Taiwan and Asia, who are looking for information on how to navigate foreign healthcare systems that do not offer information in English.

My work is well known around the world and it has been recognized by:

- *Healthline for Outstanding Fibromyalgia Blog;*
- *WEGO Health as Lifetime Achievement Award finalist for my website at MySeveralWorlds.com,;*
- *The Spondylitis Association of America for providing patients with tips and advice on living with inflammatory arthritis;*
- *I'm also a founding director for Walk AS One, which is a 501c3 non profit organization that was established in 2016.*

Ankylosing spondyloarthritis derailed my life because it took so long to get a diagnosis and then there was a delay to treatment, but this takes us back around to the start of my story.

Life is a journey and I have journeyed long and hard. The experiences – good and bad - are all part of the process. When life decided to take me on a journey with chronic illness, I went with it just like I went with all the adventures I've had with travel. Although I've had to give up things I love the most, I found other things that I love equally as much. I've found other ways to live life to the fullest, and my story today is really what life is all about.

Some things never go according to plans. Some things go just as you expected. And some things bring you right to where you belong, and I do believe that my journey has brought me right here where I belong in life, living a full life in Asia and loving it.

My travels have helped me gain perspective on life. In the midst of illness, I could still choose how I wanted to live each day within my limits and who I wanted to be. I used to be a traveler, but now my days are filled with helping others navigate their own journeys. And we can take those journeys together. After all, the point is to keep moving forward.

We bend, we don't break. We keep on going.

Jennifer Blair

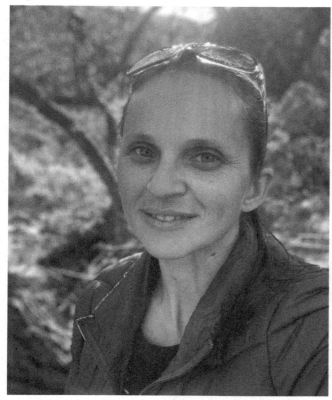

"I have always had the mentality of "keep going." It's just something my brain did when I was young."

One morning I woke up with a swollen ankle. My parents thought I may have gotten it caught in my crib, so they took me to the doctor to be safe. The doctor told my mom and dad, "she has juvenile rheumatoid arthritis." My parents were shocked to hear that. I was only one years old and had a lifetime of challenges coming my way, socially, physically, mentally and emotionally.

I was started on medication right away. Quickly followed by weekly blood tests, physical therapy and monthly doctor's visits. By the time I was in elementary school I was told that I was depressed. Of course I was, I was in almost constant physical pain everyday of my life. At school I would crawl on my knees to the pencil sharpener because it hurt so much to walk. My meds would occasionally change and cause me to fall asleep in class. When I would arrive at school, I would be in so much pain I would go to the nurses office and just lay on one of those old school beds they had back then. I was hospitalized twice, once when I was nine and once at age eleven.

When I was nine years old my knees started to stay at a bent angle and wouldn't straighten, and of course I was in pain. I couldn't walk like that so the doctor decided to have my legs cereal casted for a month to fuse them straight. It was horrible. Every four days I would come into the hospital and they would push my knees straight and cast them all the way up to my thighs. One time, a person who had never removed a cast before decided to cut my casts off. This was before the small vibrating saw they now have to remove casts. You know the one that just tickles. This one did not tickle. This saw was much bigger and sharp. As the lady started to cut through my casts I started to scream and tell them it was cutting me. She told me and my parents, "it's just warm." I was then held down by several people until she cut through both casts, then removed them from my legs. I was bleeding about every four inches from my thigh to my ankle on both sides of both of my legs. My mom just walked away crying. It was a horrible experience. I cried so much and now realized how in that moment my voice didn't matter.

I have taken that with me my whole life. As a child and now an adult. I still struggle to voice the things I'm thinking and feeling. I struggle to be secure in my own body and to speak up for myself. It's a struggle to love who and how I am. It's a huge struggle to fight against all the negative thoughts and self deprecation.

I have now had arthritis for 36 years. I have many stories of trials and victories. One of the best things I've done for myself and my body is to seriously work on my mindset. To know myself and how and why I run the way I do. I have always had the mentality of "keep going." It's just something my brain did when I was young. Having a strong mindset has helped me so much in my life. To push through pain and not let it take over is a battle, for me a daily battle. I mean, I have felt physical pain every single day of my life. It's a fight mentally, physically and emotionally, as they are all intertwined. It's a fight to know in my mind that my body does not define me. It's a fight to feel the physical pain and to keep going (but I do). It's a fight to feel all the emotions that come with the pain of arthritis.

Having JRA has made me the person I am today. It has given me the drive to always keep going. Each struggle has taught me something and has a purpose. I can do anything. Watch me.

Rollin Johnson Jr.

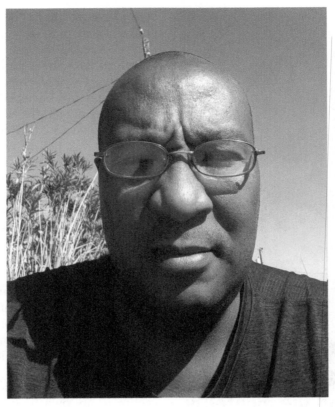

"Try and manage this to the best of your ability, use pain management as well, that's what I am gonna do. Good luck."

Probably diagnosed with arthritis back while I was in the service in the 1990's. I always blew it off because I was in my 20's and didn't know any better. In 2007 I was diagnosed with OA. I then was given pain pills and steroid injections every four months. There was no relief from either one. Many years later in 2020 I was injured on the job, mostly due to having OA instability in my knees. I ended up tearing my meniscus on the medial side and there were lateral tears as well. I had surgery to remove 20% of my meniscus. After surgery and some physical therapy I thought about going back to work. Well little did I know the surgery caused my OA to be a lot worse.

I couldn't stand or sit in one place for more than 3/4 hours without pain starting to hurt on the inside of both knees.

I now have mild osteoarthritis in both knees. Mentally, physically and emotionally this is troublesome. How are we supposed to survive if we are in too much pain to work a normal job or physical labor or whatever? We then may get addicted to pain pills and whatever else there is for us to deal with. It's very depressing when you're used to providing for yourself and know you barely have the means to survive on your own anymore. I do not wish any kind of arthritis on anyone at all. But as the saying goes only the strong survive right? How is it possible to work or rely on people's generosity? That gets old after a while.

Samantha Moss

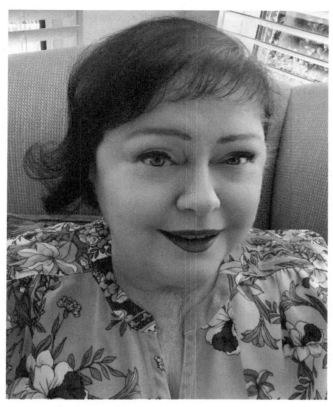

"Learning to live life differently and well with a sudden change in life's direction, particularly due to a disability, can be extremely difficult. It's so important to remember life is more than any chronic illness. We are more than our diseases."

A Case of Chronic Illness Overload

You know how it feels to be watching a really sad movie, or reading an emotionally charged book and you just need a break from it. Well, at the moment, I feel the same writing about my rheumatoid arthritis story. I'm feeling a little sick of my complex chronic illness. I need to push pause, change the channel, read another book. Not forever, just for a moment.

I medically retired in January 2014 due to a complex medical history, which can be best summed up as an overarching idiopathic disease. It includes rheumatoid arthritis and a rare idiopathic bone disease, causing widespread pathological bone fractures and severe spinal stenosis, among other things.

Living with a disability of any kind can be incredibly challenging. Learning to live life differently and well with a sudden change in life's direction, particularly due to a disability, can be extremely difficult.

Life is more than any chronic illness. I am more than my disease.

However, as the years go by, I feel more and more defined as the chronic illness blogger/writer, who runs an online support forum for others living with the same reality. Yes, it's true. It's who I am, it's what I do and what I live with everyday.

It's only a part of me though and I think I'm even losing sight of the real me, as I am engulfed with my pain and the pain of others. I'm clearly having a case of "Chronic Illness Overload" and I'm pretty sure I'm not alone. So I need to solve this if I'm going to be effective in my desire to help others and not lose myself in a chronic illness cavern.

We all know the saying "too much of a good thing." Well, it's very possible to also have too much of a bad thing. No matter the extremes of life, the good and the bad, we need a rest. Periods of amazing happiness or excitement have their use by date. We have to return to a level of normalcy where life is on an even keel. Always looking for the next adventure and injection of excitement is not sustainable, or even conducive to healthy well being.

It's the same with focusing on the hard realities of life like a chronic illness. You have to switch off at some point and try to be normal. Try and remember who you are underneath the layers of symptoms and diagnoses.

If I feel fatigued by my own story, I can't help but imagine how others must feel reading about it. Even the progression and updates must be causing stress and an overarching sense of needing to change the channel.

Members on my online support forum often feel hurt by the response, or lack of, from friends and family when they share medical news. Let's consider though, these people do care and are concerned and love you, but they can only take so much too. It's entirely feasible they have a case of chronic illness overload and need to push pause, take a break, turn the page, and listen to another story.

The Other Me, The Other You
- So, chronic illness aside, who are you, who am I?
- I'm a wife who dearly loves her husband;
- I'm passionate about interior decorating and love my home;
- I'm a singer and love music;
- I'm a friend who will always support and love those closest to her;
- I love road trips in the countryside;
- I love garden cafes with gift stores attached;
- I was a Leader in the business world for 30 years and am still passionate about leading and coaching as opportunities present;
- I love change management;
- I love writing, non fiction is my main passion. I've studied freelance journalism and non fiction writing and my memoirs, "My Medical Musings, a Story of Love, Laughter, Faith and Hope; Living with a Rare Disease," has just been published;
- I love accounting. I've always had a love of numbers and partially completed a Diploma of Accounting for fun! So creating budgets, cash flow projections, managing accounts, is my idea of a good time;
- I'm a Christian, who loves God, and my faith is my life foundation;
- I'm far from perfect. I get grumpy, I can shout and rant with the best of them, but I never hold a grudge and will say sorry first, within an hour usually. I hate being/staying angry;
- I love murder mystery TV shows, period/historical dramas and You Tube French chateau renovation channels;
- I love studying history;
- I love flowers, especially roses;
- I love entertaining at home, although nowadays I can only cope with one or two visitors, for morning or afternoon tea;
- I'm passionate about helping others;
- I'm a clean freak and make no apology for it;
- I love makeup, clothes and making myself look as nice as possible;
- I love road trips and holidaying at home in Australia. I love my country;
- I love sending greeting cards and I save any received;
- I love wrapping presents;
- I love collecting teapots, pretty mugs and plates and clocks.

Connections Are Important
If you are reading this and feeling weighed down with your own case of chronic illness overload, take some time to reconnect with who you really are. What would your "who am I list" look like?

If you are a friend or loved one of someone with chronic illness and are also experiencing a case of chronic illness overload, it's okay, we get it!

Perhaps connect with your friend or loved one, by letting them know you're overwhelmed and you'd love to do something, with them or for them, non health related.

So let's dump our case of chronic illness overload and realize it's so important to feel connected with who we are, aside from our diseases, and with others in our lives who are so important to us. We are all so much more than our chronic illness!

Patrice Johnson

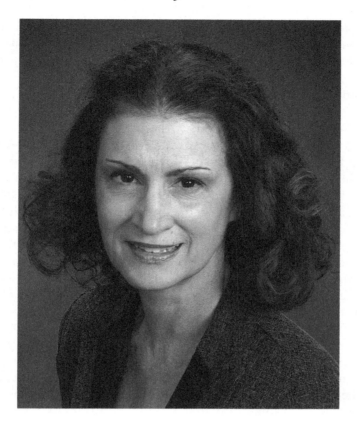

"The emotional and mental aspect of living with an incurable and chronic disease."

My story begins when I was between 12 and 13 years old. I sustained a traumatic injury to my left knee, followed by two surgeries to repair the significant damage. This ended my career as a promising ballet dancer, as I had just been accepted to a ballet company.

When I was 30 years old, I began to experience great pain in this knee and was diagnosed with osteoarthritis. I was told by the doctor the only way to correct the arthritis was to have a knee replacement. He also told me that I would have to have knee replacements done every 15 years, which meant at least five more surgeries if I lived

into my 90's. Keep in mind that this was the early 1980's when there were not many treatments available for knee arthritis. I also had two young children and had no one to take care of me and the children because my husband was not (and is still not) a 50/50 partner.

Today at age 66, my knee is bone on bone. My rheumatologist always asks me when I am going to have a knee replacement and I always tell him when I am ready. And I still don't have anyone to take care of me because I am still married to the same person. He holds the health insurance and I couldn't financially manage my arthritis without health insurance.

In 2011, I was diagnosed with rheumatoid arthritis and polymyalgia rheumatica, or PMR for short. The first few years of living with RA were difficult, but the last few years I have been in remission off and on. I now manage my RA with diet, exercise, medication, and a positive attitude. Over the last 11 years, I have been through several rheumatologists, and my current one is wonderful. (Rheumy #1 retired, and I fired rheumy #2 and #3.)

In 2020 I was diagnosed with OA in my hands, hips, spine and lower back. Having OA in these joints is a daily struggle for me. I have good days and bad days. In addition to my OA and RA, I have had several comorbidities. I have had a vein ablation, and now have anemia, osteopenia, and severe hearing loss.

In January of 2017 I was at the lowest part of my life. I sunk into a deep depression due to my RA and several other things going on in my life. I could not turn to a professional for help because my health insurance does not cover mental health services. I tried calling several professionals in my area asking if they would see me and I would pay the out of pocket costs, but no one would agree to this. I was also not aware of the national suicide prevention number. Five years ago, mental health in arthritis patients was not something that was made aware of in the healthcare profession. I had a bottle of pills in one hand and a glass of water in the other, but when I opened the bottle of pills, something stopped me. I cannot name or describe what this was except, in my book, I think it was some kind of divine intervention. I put the bottle of pills away and tossed the glass of water. I do not remember the rest of the day.

A few weeks after coming close to ending my life, I began to volunteer for several arthritis non profit organizations. I wasn't sure I could help anyone or that anyone would even want to hear my story. Over the next few years I became extremely active in volunteering for these non profits.

Over the last several years on my arthritis journey I have dealt with out of pocket medical costs, delays in treatment, and being denied treatment.

Being an arthritis patient has actually been a blessing for me. Of course I would never wish for anyone to have any form of this disease, but for me it truly did save my life. After my RA diagnosis, my husband refused to help me emotionally or physically while living with arthritis. I then realized that no one was going to help me with my arthritis but myself. I have learned to speak up, question doctors, fight for my medical rights and always help other arthritis patients when asked. I also advocate nationally and locally for arthritis patients' rights.

Every January I reflect on how much I have had to overcome living with arthritis and not just the physical portion of it. I think this has made me a stronger person. Also having arthritis has made me more empathetic to anyone struggling and trying to live with a chronic and incurable disease. I am a better listener too. I am extremely grateful that whatever intervened for me on that dark January day, I am still here and doing what I love, helping other arthritis patients.

At the beginning of my RA diagnosis, my first rheumatologist told me that there is a 60% chance I will pass this down to my children and grandchildren. And my current rheumatologist stated that my recent OA diagnosis is due to my family ancestry, although there is no history of it in my mind. Passing RA and/or OA onto my children and five grandchildren is a heavy burden to carry and it weighs on my mind constantly.

In addition to what I already do, my goal for the future is to focus on the mental issues that so many arthritis patients face. There is a greater need for support groups, more training for rheumatologists whose patients are dealing with depression and other mental issues, and also to bring awareness that arthritis is just not dealing with physical pain. More access to mental health professionals is needed. Families, caregivers, and healthcare professionals need more education with regards to depression, anxiety and other mental health issues that we arthritis patients face every day of our lives.

In the last year or so, mental health issues in top athletes has been the topic of many media stories. This is great that a light is being shed on their struggles, but what about people living with arthritis, or any incurable disease? Why can't our mental health issues become a top priority as well?

Hannah-Rayne Plummer

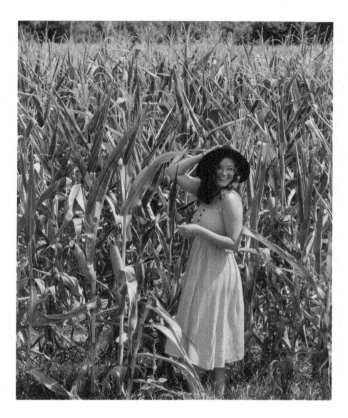

"I've come to the conclusion that I want to THRIVE. Living just to make it to the next pain filled day sounds horrible if I'm honest! I want my life to be more than my illness, diagnosis, and symptoms."

I am 21 years old, and I have been living with diagnosed chronic pain for the past three years. Before my diagnosis I experienced pain, lots of it, and hoped and prayed I'd get a simple, 'fixable', diagnosis from my doctor. Instead I was met with tests, blood work, very little answers, and even more symptoms aside from 'pain'. I received a "textbook diagnosis," because my blood work and symptoms checked all the boxes for ankylosing spondylitis. This was back in 2018. Today, in 2022, I have more symptoms than before, the same diagnosis, and an ongoing search for answers, symptom control

ideas, and a purpose in living with an invisible illness.

Something I've wrestled with over time is the phrase 'Thriving over Surviving'. What does that look like in my life? How can I help other people understand it? And do I want to thrive, or simply survive one day to the next?

I've come to the conclusion that I want to THRIVE. Living just to make it to the next pain filled day sounds horrible if I'm honest! I want my life to be more than my illness, diagnosis, and symptoms. So how do I make this happen? There are tons of ways to make this easier but I wanted to share three things with you that help me enter a THRIVE mindset.

- **Acceptance** - This one is HARD. But when I decided to accept my diagnosis and make it a part of my life, my day to day became so much easier! I learned what food affected my body and made the necessary changes. I figured out the best clothes to help me feel comfortable and supported. I got a new mattress to help me sleep better, etc. When we accept our illness as a part of our future then we can make the changes necessary to make that future something to look forward to!
- **Community** - Something that helps me MAJORLY, when it comes to wanting to do more than just survive the bad days, is finding people who understand what I am going through and who are going through it with me! Whether this is people with a similar diagnosis, friends who are willing to learn about my illness, or a blog, vlog, or podcast about my illness that I can relate to. Having friends I can vent to, complain to, process with, or encourage one another, makes THRIVING so much easier because the bad days aren't so lonely! Bad days come, when 'surviving' is the best I can do, but having people around me who I can share those bad days with makes a huge difference!
- **Goals** - Mini goals, from getting out of bed with my alarm, to Big goals, like moving out of my mom's house and everything in between. When I make goals I find myself feeling more productive, more positive and more willing to keep going with my day. A simple 'cross off the list' or 'check the box' can feel SO GOOD because it lets us know we did it! And it's time to move to the next thing. This helps my day feel less mundane and helps those flare days feel less drowsy and lazy. Celebrate the little victories because you are doing GREAT! Even on the hard days.

I hope any of these three things can help you, encourage you, or relate to you so you don't feel so alone! Chronic illness, pain, and invisible symptoms are SCARY, HARD, and SUCK. I know what you are going through! So if you felt alone in any way... YOU ARE NOT ALONE ANYMORE. Accept your diagnosis as part of your life, find a community to support you, and set up some easy goals because this life is about SO much more than simply getting through the next 80 years. Thrive! Don't let arthritis kick your butt, YOU KICK ARTHRITIS' BUTT instead! Beautiful human, you are worthy of a great life.

Emily Theis

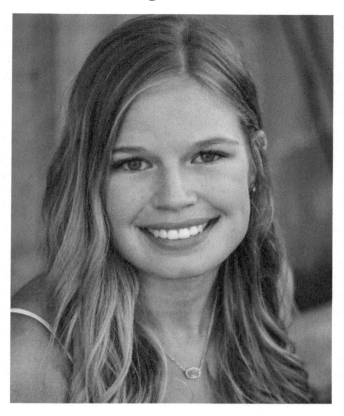

Just because I have arthritis doesn't mean I can't do things just like everyone else. I have proved to not only myself, but also everyone else that I can do amazing things."

One thing that most people don't realize is that while having juvenile arthritis is a physical disease, it often tends to take quite a toll on a person mentally as well. There are many times in my life I felt alone, anxious, and scared. It all started in about fourth grade when suddenly one day I realized I couldn't move as well as I usually could. Over time it continued to get worse and I could barely walk or write. Eventually, my parents noticed and took me to my pediatrician. We were told that I was just having growing pains and to take over the counter pain medicine whenever I felt I needed it.

I was still in constant pain and continued to get worsening symptoms. I went from being one of the most athletic kids in my class to barely being able to walk.

We went back to the pediatrician multiple times and got blood tests done but they couldn't figure out why I was in such pain. I knew something more was wrong with me but no one seemed to believe me but my parents. The pain got to the point where I never wanted to do anything because it hurt so bad. I didn't want to go to school, I didn't want to hang out with my friends. All I wanted to do was lay in bed. Teachers and staff at the school began to notice the change in my behavior. They thought I was going into depression as I never wanted to eat much either. My mom and dad continued to take me to the pediatrician, and he finally referred me to Children's Hospital in Omaha to see a rheumatologist. At Children's Hospital, the doctor diagnosed me with juvenile idiopathic arthritis at my first appointment. I started taking pain management medications that immediately started to make me feel better.

Everything should have gotten better, considering that I wasn't in so much pain, but finding out I had arthritis only seemed to complicate things even more. I was constantly worried about what my friends would think of me if they found out I had arthritis. I was worried that they would make fun of me since arthritis is supposed to be an "elderly" disease. I kept my diagnosis a secret for about six months. Telling my friends that I had arthritis ultimately was the best decision I'd ever made. My friends supported me and would always check in on me to see how I was doing. I was also going to physical and occupational therapy at this time and enjoyed going. At times it was challenging, but I couldn't wait to be able to do all the things I used to do easily again.

I became quite frustrated because I graduated from physical therapy before I graduated from occupational therapy. I was mad at myself because writing was one of the most difficult things for me to relearn how to do. I was able to take this anger and use it as a drive to work on writing more at home, so I could be completely done with therapy.

All was finally good, until about sixth grade when I had my first flare up. I got really down on myself as I felt like I had finally figured out how to go about normal day to day things with my arthritis. Since I had a flare up my rheumatologist decided to put me on methotrexate injections. This was really scary to me as I was afraid of needles. Every Wednesday night, when it was time to get my injection, my mom and dad would have to chase me downstairs in order to give it to me. I grew to hate my parents for making me have this injection, I mean what kid wants to have to get a shot every week. I didn't understand it at the time but all my parents wanted for me was to help me get better. Eventually, my mom and dad helped me learn how to give myself shots. I liked to give myself shots as it helped me feel more in control of everything that was going on around me.

Fast forward to high school, everything was great. Sports are important in my family so my parents encouraged me to go out for every sport. Playing sports was a struggle as it was quite a love hate relationship. It's hard to find joy in doing something that just tends to make your body ache. Sometimes all I wanted to do was quit. My dad often tended to push me in sports as he knew I had potential and he loved to watch sports. It was difficult to manage all of my school work, sports practices, and arthritis. Looking back I am glad my dad pushed me so much in sports, as I am one of the lucky ones. Not everyone my age with arthritis is lucky enough to get to play sports. I had learned that after every game it helped my body to take a hot shower and relax afterwards. At this point I had realized that, yes it does suck, I have arthritis but I was making the best situation possible out of the cards life had dealt me.

This year I am a freshman in college. This has presented new struggles as I am two hours away from my family. Learning to manage my arthritis all on my own has been quite the adventure. Going to college in itself is a big life change, but having to deal with this change, all the while having arthritis, took a toll on me mentally. I realized that I couldn't handle everything all by myself and ended up going to see the mental health counselor on campus. She really helped me talk through everything that was going on in my life. She also really helped me learn to adjust to college life. At first I was embarrassed to be going to a therapist, then after talking about it with some of my friends, I realized that quite a few of them also went to therapists and that it was nothing to be ashamed of. College has been a fun adventure and I can't wait to keep making memories here.

Just because I have arthritis doesn't mean I can't do things just like everyone else. By playing sports I proved this to not only myself but also my peers. No one would've ever thought a girl with arthritis would've been able to make it to the Nebraska State Track Meet... but I did. I have learned to never let my arthritis hold me back. I can do amazing things just like everyone else if I put my mind to it.

Sophie Truepenny

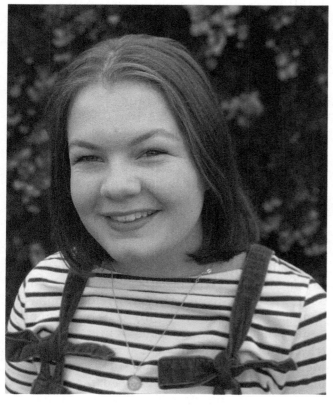

"I think it's common to feel isolated in difficult situations and to wholeheartedly believe that no one has ever experienced what you're facing. But I'm learning that people are sharing their stories, that someone, somewhere has been there before, we just have to know where to find them, and we just need to hear them. When niche stories are told we find that they're not so niche after all."

I'm an undergrad studying Zoology at the University of Cambridge, UK. Having arthritis has forced me to change the way I view myself as an individual, my 'role' in society and my communities, and the way my life will look. Let me explain how a metaphor and a little history lesson have aided this growth.

I had symptoms from around 15 years old but was not diagnosed until I was 20, by which point the diagnosis, a label, an answer, and a name for this pain, was a relief. For a while, the diagnosis gave me hope and I felt more positive about my future knowing what I was facing. But with time, what once lifted a weight from my shoulders, brought a heavy burden. In my second year of university, I became more ill and uni work, exercise, socializing and dealing with a chronic illness in a pandemic became too much. I felt isolated, I couldn't do the things I loved, and my mental health was suffering.

When mindfulness and my usual habits to lift my mood weren't enough, in an effort to help myself when I felt no one else could, I started writing poetry, in a document I had called 'sh*t coffee table poetry'. Calling it so took away any pressure I might put on myself to produce something 'worthwhile', and be productive, while I was trying to rest.

I felt like I never understood the poetry I read. Poetry from the bookshop or the school library was all war, peace, straight relationships, adult things…healthy people. And subconsciously I started to write the poetry I needed myself, that I needed to read then. The messy emotions of growing out of your teen years as a queer youth, having never been out in childhood. The weight of facing losses no one could see or console. The pressure of getting through university with chronic pain.

I was naïve to think no one understood how I felt and how I had felt. I think it's common to feel isolated in difficult situations and to wholeheartedly believe that no one has ever experienced what you're facing. But I'm learning that people are sharing their stories, that someone, somewhere has been there before, we just have to know where to find them, and we just need to hear them. When niche stories are told we find that they're not so niche after all.

When I was first coming to terms with being queer, as is the universal queer experience, I watched every coming out video on YouTube. I found all the LGBTQ+ TV shows and I read all the queer stories I could. I learned so much not only about myself, but also about this amazing community I was growing into. Queer representation in media and films (and poetry), was and still is hard to find, and I'm a white, English speaking, mostly cis-presenting person. But it is abundant in comparison to the representation of disabled people.

When I got diagnosed with psoriatic arthritis (PsA), I did exactly the same thing. I did so much research; I watched every video, I followed every hashtag on Instagram, and I learned everything I could about this new community I had suddenly become a part of. But there wasn't enough. As far as I knew, other people had it bad, worse than I, and all the time that wasn't true for me. I considered myself lucky that I was still able to play ice hockey, I could still go to uni, I was still happy. I was in pain all the time, yes, but for a while, I was still living.

There were a few big things that little bit of representation didn't prepare me for: the ups and downs, the admin and the pacing. Writing poetry helped me to find a metaphor to come to terms with my PsA.

If a healthy person's life is a walk in the park with arthritis, life is a hike in the mountains. From their well-trodden paths, some appreciate that life is more difficult for us up here - 'you have a tough climb,'I can see that you're struggling, you have further to go'.

Some offer to help - 'can we carry anything for you?'.

Some even think our treacherous journey is better - 'but you get such good views from up there' or 'I'd love to stay in bed all day' and 'it must be nice to spend longer in the sun' or 'you're lucky, you get extensions and disability perks'.

The weather on this mountain is all over the place. Unpredictable. Ever-changing. The fog is perhaps the most annoying. We don't know where we're going, what's next, how we'll cope. One day we'll struggle to take a few steps, but the next we'll be laughing and chatting as we scale a steep part of the climb. While I knew that having this condition would make life more complicated, I didn't expect that my days and 'the weather' would be so variable. Often, I struggle to get up in the mornings because of my pain, but by the evening, when 'the fog has cleared', I can usually exercise. The variability in and between days is something I'm still coming to terms with. When I'm doing well, I assume it isn't as bad as I think, but when I'm not doing well, I struggle to remember the good times.

And while for a walk in the park you don't need to plan, or tell anyone where you're going, or take anything with you, a hike or a climb in the mountains is another level

Whoever said having a chronic illness is like a full-time job was right. What started as an appointment every few months quickly turned into biweekly bloods, chasing prescriptions, constant telephone calls and check-ups. It's like climbing without a map, trying to make your own map without anything to make it with and then watching it crumble in the rain.

Thinking about my PsA like this reminds me to stop comparing myself to people around me and has helped me make some big decisions in favor of my health.

One of my favorite lessons from history comes from the story of the race to the South Pole, which reminds me of the importance of pacing (spreading out and limiting daily activities to not exacerbate one's condition).

Roald Amundsen led the Norwegian team to the South Pole in a race against Robert Scott's British team. They each took opposing approaches, leading to wildly different outcomes - only one team returned. While the British traveled as much as they could each day, with the focus of the expedition being simply to reach the pole first, the Norwegians paced themselves. It is said that on the days with bad conditions, the Norwegians would aim to cover 15 nautical miles, but on the days with good weather conditions, the team would limit themselves to the same distance of 15 nautical miles. Not only did Amundsen's team beat Scotts to the pole by 33 days, but they had the strength and resources to complete the return journey.

A lot can be learned from Amundsen's success; I think of this story when I am struggling to pace myself. With daily tasks, it can be useful to set both lower and upper limits on activities. It is perhaps easier said than done, but on the good days, don't do too much, and on the bad days, still do a little. Pacing is the most sustainable way to achieve our goals, it might even get us there faster.

Limiting ourselves is hard, and it can be lonely up on our peaks. Finding my community of young people with arthritis through the UK charity, Versus Arthritis, has been another invaluable tool for coping with this disease, and I will be forever grateful that I have people on this hike with me.

We gain a lot of perspective from these climbs, but it never makes the next one easier. Though most mornings I have trouble getting out of bed, writing is the one thing I can always turn to. When I'm in pain, in bed and alone, I read or add to my 'sh*t coffee table poetry' and imagine myself somewhere on a foggy mountain, or maybe an Antarctic glacier.

I hope having read this, and the other stories in this collection, that you feel less alone, or that you understand more and we can find each other somewhere in these mountains. I will forever fight for future media to show more of how beautiful and difficult it can be to live (and love) as we do, and as there is no cure, this is the hill I will die on.

Chelsea Flores

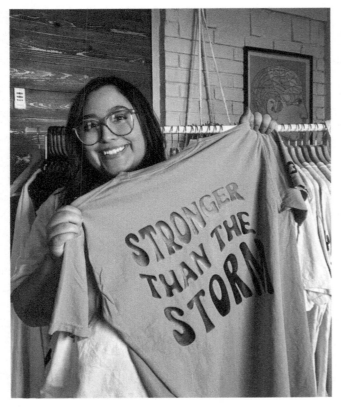

"Stronger than the Storm."

I am the Co-Owner of Juniper and Wildflower. I was diagnosed with rheumatoid arthritis three years ago at 24. I had just received my undergrad, started my new job and had only been married for three months when I received my diagnosis. I had this vision of what my life would look like at that time and it quickly vanished. Since learning of my autoimmune disease, my life has changed drastically. I had to quit my job because the company was unwilling to accommodate my health needs. I dropped out of grad school because I didn't have the mental capacity to add the stress of school to my plate. And if that wasn't enough, my physical appearance was changing, my relationships started to look different and my mental health deteriorated. I had no idea what my future held.

When I learned of my RA, I knew the battle would be challenging physically, but I didn't realize how damaging it would be to my mental health. I didn't think I would have to say goodbye to my old self. I felt like the life I had worked so hard for was gone. I couldn't see past the storm.

As time went on, the anxiety, depression, and suicidal thoughts increased. I've never felt more lonely than when I had to try to navigate my new "normal." I felt like I had to take on this journey alone, have the best support system through my family and my husband, Angel. I found it challenging to explain to them the pain I endured or the emotional suffering I was experiencing. So, I decided to survive on my own for fear of burdening my family. I tried to hide my anxiety, the panic attacks, the anger, and the constant tears behind a smile. It wasn't until my 27th birthday that I hit rock bottom.

I was at the lowest I'd ever been. My flares were constant, I developed scleritis in my right eye and I was experiencing hair loss. I remember looking in the mirror one day and I could not recognize the person looking back at me. The week leading up to my birthday, Angel had to force me out of bed. I'd cry every day for hours and spend most of my time on the couch watching TV. I felt like my life was in constant chaos, so I tried to distract myself because I wasn't sure how much longer I could go on. My diagnosis broke my faith, and I was numb to the world. It was at this point that I had to seek help. I finally decided to go to therapy.

I was diagnosed with depression, anxiety, and PTSD. I remember telling my therapist that I don't know who I am anymore. She responded, *"it's okay that you don't know. We will work on helping you remember who you are and who you are becoming."* That sentence was the light bulb moment for me.

I needed to grieve my past life to be able to move on. I am learning that if I stay angry and hold on to the past, I remain stuck. And I am learning to take healing into my own hands by having grace for myself. Although my self-healing journey has just begun, I know that 24-year-old me is proud of how far I've come. She would be proud of the steps I'm choosing to take to heal and be vulnerable. I am still learning to love myself, but I am finding power in the woman I am becoming. I am not a broken shell of a person because of my diagnosis. And as I continue to take steps forward in this journey, I know that I am stronger than the storm.

Analisa Politano

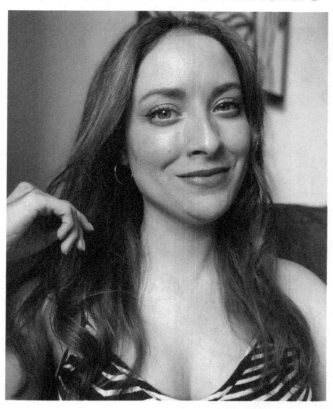

"Perspective is everything."

Perspective is everything. I believe it was Albert Einstein who once said, *"There are two ways to live your life. One is as though nothing is a miracle. The other is as though everything is a miracle."* Over the years, many people have commended me on my "great positive attitude" throughout my chronic illness journey. Unfortunately, I don't think they quite understand how much willpower and strength it takes to accomplish this daily. They don't understand that I really have no other choice. If I don't push forward and take the time to truly appreciate the little things life has to offer, I can easily go into a negative downward spiral. In the past, I've been in that dark place and tried not to fall down the rabbit hole.

Rheumatoid arthritis and other chronic illnesses cause a great deal of loss and inconsistencies. It affects every aspect of my waking life. In my world, I'm consistently inconsistent because of all the disruptions due to my illnesses. As a result, I feel the only thing I can truly control is my mind frame.

Something I make sure I do daily is to observe and absorb the beauty the sky has to offer. I can't tell you how many pictures of the sunrises and sunsets I have saved. This little act helps calm my mind, as I remember all the good that surrounds me. Many people laugh because they say I act like Brendan Fraser's character in Bedazzled, who cries over the beauty of the sunset and yes, that's me. These illnesses have taught me to stop and appreciate the little things.

You have the choice every day to choose your perspective in life. I can easily be negative everyday but what would that accomplish? Negativity affects your mind, body, spirit, people around you and more. You can't just ignore your illnesses but you can help yourself mentally by appreciating all the things you do have. My life still holds lots more beauty, laughs, and personal development. This is how I have chosen to view my world and is what keeps me going. I hope to inspire at least one person to change their perspective and be more aware of the little things in life.

Dina Pittman

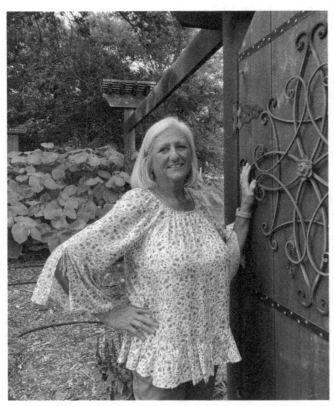

"Don't let the word JUST hijack the prognosis for your arthritis!"

It's Not JUST Arthritis
AKA The Disabled Gardener

You've been struggling with physical things lately. Increasingly you need help. Your joints are swollen, you're losing energy to keep up with the things you used to do all day long.

Your doctor runs tests. You spend a few weeks anxious about the results, and then they finally return with the results and jovially claim, "No worries, it's JUST arthritis."

Has this been your experience? It was mine and it changed the course of my life. Saying "it's JUST arthritis" has had a serious impact on my mental health since my diagnosis. I don't mean to paint the doctor as a bad person. Maybe they were JUST relieved they didn't have to tell me

I was dying and the alternative of JUST having arthritis was great news! But that word JUST is an UNJUST word!

It's JUST arthritis.
JUST take Ibuprofen.
JUST lose weight.
JUST stop gardening.
It's JUST normal aging.

One quarter of the population has arthritis. That's a lot of people! It's typically thought of as the old person's disease. Something everyone will eventually get. The wear and tear disease. All those things can be true, but there's so much more to it. Using the word JUST to describe osteoarthritis makes it less than for the person receiving the diagnosis and creates a burden of guilt and shame.

Was I supposed to be happy that I have osteoarthritis in every joint in my body? Was I the cause of my osteoarthritis because I'm overweight? Because I overused my joints? Because I garden? Because I'm aging? Was I the cause of my own pain?

Without realizing it, I was allowing others to blame me for this disease.

When I asked why I have such bad osteoarthritis, I was told I'd been hard on my body. When I asked what I can do about osteoarthritis pain, I was told to take ibuprofen.

When I asked about my prognosis for the future, I got the mixed message that there's nothing you can do about it, everyone gets it. Wait. Was I the cause of my arthritis? Or is it inevitable?

The truth is, osteoarthritis is a complex disease, without a cure. Research is revealing more about it all the time, throwing new light on the causes.

When people say it's JUST arthritis, it steals your ability to make a positive change in your prognosis.

But the worst part is when you tell yourself it's JUST arthritis. The problem and the solution are easy. You JUST have wear and tear on your joints due to age, weight, and overuse so, JUST lose weight, JUST stop gardening, JUST take Ibuprofen. Easy right?

Researchers are finding that the problem isn't all wear and tear. Overuse and age can add to the development of osteoarthritis, but many more factors beyond our control are at play like joint injury, musculoskeletal abnormalities, genetics, weak muscles, gender, and environmental factors.

Combinations of these factors and hormonal issues can make it difficult to lose weight and the cycle of pain makes it hard to exercise. Gardening is the activity that brings me joy. It's what I'm most passionate about and provides me with an emotional, physical, and creative outlet. Telling me to JUST stop gardening is devastating!

Daily ibuprofen was causing stomach issues and it has a list of negative long-term effects. I needed a better way to manage my osteoarthritis! But if I continued to buy the line it's JUST arthritis, I was powerless to do anything about it. The only way to get my power back was to say, "Enough!" It's not JUST arthritis any more than I'm not JUST a gardener.

Osteoarthritis is a serious disease of the joints that for a variety of intertwined reasons has manifested its way into my life. It's a disease that medical science doesn't have a cure for, but one that I can learn to manage.

And so, I'm learning to reinvent myself from someone who JUST has arthritis, to someone who's doing something about it. I've developed my own management plan for my arthritis. One that will let me continue to pursue my passion for gardening for the rest of my life in a way that allows for healthy aging for arthritic joints.

My management program, the Pillars of Strength, has six pillars that are integral to each other.

The six pillars are:

1. *Mind-Management* – Manage the way I'm thinking about my arthritis, starting with removing the word JUST! I have osteoarthritis, a serious disease of the joints. Through integrated management, I can pursue my passions and dreams in life, despite arthritis. I didn't cause osteoarthritis, but I can choose to have a positive effect on my prognosis.

2. *Exercise* – I can find or develop exercise programs that cater to my specific joint problems and help strengthen me to compensate for the weak areas of my body. It has taken some mind management to convince myself that I'm a person who loves to exercise! But I do it for the love of my joints and my desire to continue gardening.

3. *Nutrition* – I'm discovering that what I eat directly affects how I feel. Sugar is a major player in creating inflammation in the body, as is gluten. I use the garden to gradually replace my love for refined carbs with a love for fresh fruits and vegetables. Some supplements can have a positive effect on my pain levels long-term and are a great alternative to daily Ibuprofen. I'm becoming more aware that what I put in my body has a significant impact on pain and inflammation. Like creating a great environment for plants to grow in the garden, I need to create a positive biome for healing in my body.

4. *Methods* – I research new gardening methods constantly, to find ways to garden that impact my joints the least but create a beautiful impact on my life. Gone are my old back-breaking ways. I'm constantly on the search for better gardening methods that allow me to nurture both the garden and my body.

5. *Tools* – Simple changes like replacing a wheelbarrow with a garden cart, regular pruners with ratcheting pruners and metal watering cans with plastic, are easy solutions to overworking joints. I'm re-thinking all the tools I use and making sure they work harder for me.

6. *Pain Relief* – With arthritis there's going to be pain. I must give myself grace on days when I need it. Self-care is paramount and I can't let it slide. I'm finding alternative means of pain relief, knowing that it may not be one but a combination of several things I can use regularly to provide pain relief for aching joints.

With these six pillars, I know I can create an unbreakable foundation for living my life my way with arthritis. It's my choice. I can believe it's JUST arthritis, something not to be taken seriously. JUST keep pushing it under and try to ignore what it's doing to my body. JUST take the Ibuprofen and continue to feel guilty for what I've caused and shame that I won't JUST lose weight. JUST sweep it under the rug as if it isn't creating life-altering differences. Everyone gets it right? It must be ravaging everyone else's lives too.

Or I can say, enough. I have arthritis and I intend to learn everything I can to find ways to manage it positively.

I hope my story helps you make a better choice for you. It's not JUST arthritis, it's your life.

Gladys Munguia

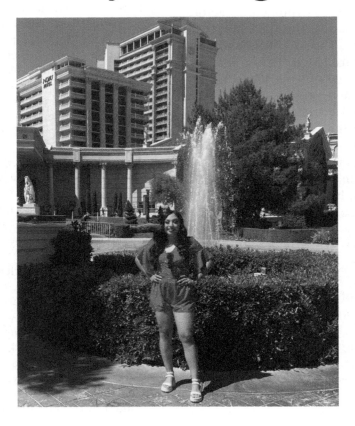

"I am learning that it is okay not to be ok, and I can still live a healthy life while having RA."

I was diagnosed with RA in 2019 at 23 years of age. I was a person who loved running, hiking, walking, dancing, working out and overall being active in every way. Getting the news that I was going to have joint pain for the rest of my life was very difficult to accept. I would never be able to have a day without pain. I spent weeks crying, being angry, wondering why at the age of 23, I was diagnosed with a disease that would affect every aspect of my life for the rest of my life.

I was so young, I was in college and still had so much to live for. I had never heard of rheumatoid arthritis before. I knew there was arthritis, but I thought that was only a thing older people got. I did not know how to deal with this diagnosis and tried to act like everything was fine. My boyfriend, now husband, was supportive every step of the way. He assured me that we would get through it.

I went an entire year post-diagnosis where I was still able to do most things. I was constantly having specialist appointments and constantly getting blood drawn. My diagnosis was all I could think about every day and night. I would spend my nights crying because I just couldn't believe that I had RA. I refused to tell anyone about it because nobody would understand. I started thinking that my boyfriend at the time was better off being with someone else because why would he want to be with someone who will eventually not be able to do most things. I was still having a hard time accepting my fate. I became very irritable, emotional and started having mood swings because I just wanted to have a day where I didn't feel pain. I no longer knew what it was like to be able to do anything and everything without any physical pain. My mental health declined and I began having emotional breakdowns, almost every month.

As more time passed, the pain in my joints moved to other parts of my body. It started with my hands, then moved to my feet, and eventually went up to my knees. In 2020, my boyfriend and I got married on Valentine's day. That day, I couldn't walk in heels that I used to be able to wear with no issue. I blamed me for not wearing heels in a while, rather than accepting it was due to my RA. I couldn't grasp the idea of eventually needing to take medication every day for the rest of my life. For an entire year, I was able to maintain my pain without medication. After the first year and a half, in June 2021, I decided to officially get on medication because the pain was becoming too much.

Once I got my prescriptions, it all hit me again that my life was changing. I started thinking about my future and everything I would have to accommodate. I do not have kids yet and I already felt like an older lady. I would think to myself, "How could I ever care for a child when I can't do much of what I used to do?." I once again spent my time crying and being angry because I had to deal with this. I would think, "Was I really a terrible person that God gave me this diagnosis?" I have never really been religious, but I assumed I was not a good person and God gave me this for a reason.

I was waking up every morning not being able to walk correctly or move my hands. On some mornings I would be so upset that my legs, feet and hands hurt, that I would break down in the middle of getting ready for work. Even though it had been two years since my diagnosis, I was upset because I just wanted to be able to wake up without any pain. I wanted to be able to do everything I was able to do before my RA diagnosis and I hated that this was my life now. I was not happy with anything in my life and I would become upset at my husband, because he didn't understand what I was going through, even though it was not his fault.

In late 2021 my feet would now be in so much pain that I would limp every time I walked. I still never really told anyone about my condition because nobody would really understand what it is, and if they did, their response would be "but you're so young!" I could no longer run more than a mile without not being able to walk the next day. I couldn't go on hikes anymore or go on long walks like I used to. I've recently had to stop going to the gym because my flare ups were becoming unbearable. There have been days where I can't even walk or have a hard time getting up when I am laying down or sitting down. Even though it has been three years since I've been diagnosed, there are times where I still feel helpless because I can't do what I wish I could. I still constantly think that my husband doesn't deserve a wife who, a lot of times, can barely walk and go dancing, hiking, or go on long walks. It is a constant physical battle, but most definitely it is more of a mental/emotional battle, having to wake up every day and be in pain.

On days that my pain is minimal, I feel happier because I can walk and do activities without issue. On days where I have flare ups, I struggle a bit more mentally because my negative thoughts take over. I am still learning new ways that I can continue to live a normal life. I am learning to accept that some days I will not be able to move at my full potential, but that is okay. I am becoming more open to letting people know and answering any questions they have regarding my experience with RA.

I am lucky to have my husband in my life, who tries to be informed on how things will affect me and is understanding on days where my flare ups don't allow me to do some things. He helps me on days that I can't do things and has been supportive throughout this entire journey. I am learning that it is okay not to be ok, and I can still live a healthy life while having RA and I will continue to find ways to continue doing what I love.

Cristal Byrns-Cavallaro

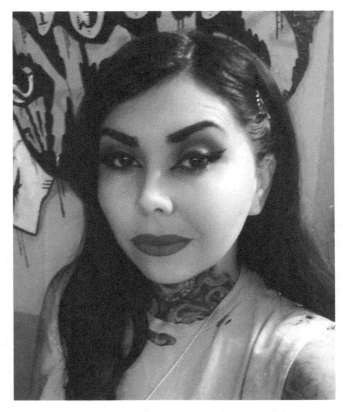

"YOU ARE NOT ALONE!"

Rheumatoid arthritis has changed my life in some ways. I went from a successful working mom of two, to having a mini stroke and being focused to quit and become a stay at home mom. Trust me! It also was a blessing in disguise I didn't realize obviously until now. My story is like many. It took almost five years of medical gaslighting until someone took me seriously, stopped telling me it was in my head and started taking the correct steps to find the root cause. At this point my toes and fingers were basically unusable and I had no idea how to handle it.

I went to so many different types of doctors until I found my neurologist and for him I'm so thankful. He took the correct steps to get me the help I needed. He referred me to a rheumatologist and after about a year of trial and error with different types of medication, I finally found something that worked. My life was finally normal or what I call normal. The thing with RA is your body is always fighting itself and it becomes tiring and frustrating for us. For example, I'm switching my biologics because my body is now fighting off my current medication.

RA is a constant battle with your body, mind and soul. You need to remember this shall pass. If today I don't feel 100%, tomorrow I might feel 10 times better. My word of advice is join a support group on Facebook, or follow RA pages to find support because you need to be around people that understand you. And the most important thing to never forget YOU ARE NOT ALONE.

Amy Burford

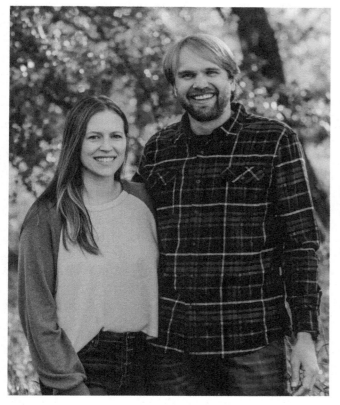

"But here I am, full of heartache and fear, still moving forward."

Getting diagnosed with rheumatoid arthritis knocked me off my feet. My RA was confirmed in the Spring of 2021, after months of doctor's appointments and persistent joint pain. The physical pain was challenging to deal with but the emotional f****** turmoil that comes along with an autoimmune disorder, still has me reeling. I did not check all the boxes for a typical RA patient so my onset was met with various versions of, *"I think it's just temporary!"* from physicians. But the pain didn't go away. And my hope that I was experiencing some weird, short-term illness dissipated.

I was overwhelmed with grief while trying to come to terms with my condition. I grieved the life I lived before my diagnosis. I grieved about the future I thought I was going to have. Learning that I would be sick forever felt like a monumental loss. My health was precious and now it's gone. I was, and still am, surprised at how much it affects my identity. I lived 35 years as a healthy person and now...I'm a sick person? I struggle with saying it out loud that I have rheumatoid arthritis. Even more so with people who I consider close. People tend to ask questions that I don't really want to answer. Those questions usually feel invasive. I'd rather not talk about how or why I think this happened. My days are speckled with reminders of my arthritis - an ache in my knees, the hair loss from my medication, or my noticeable lack of energy. Some days, on a good day, I almost feel like my old self. But I know I will never actually feel like my old self. It's easy to feel lost when you wake up in a body that no longer feels like your own. Like an unwelcome visitor has decided to move into my house. A permanent change that is invisible to everyone else, all-consuming to me.

The last year has been a struggle. It has been a year of just surviving. Many days were lived, void of enthusiasm. I think about healing often. I wonder if there has been any emotional repair in the period since my diagnosis. Can you ever heal if you are chronically ill? It feels impossible right now. But here I am, full of heartache and fear, still moving forward. And that has to count for something.

Ruth Hollingsworth

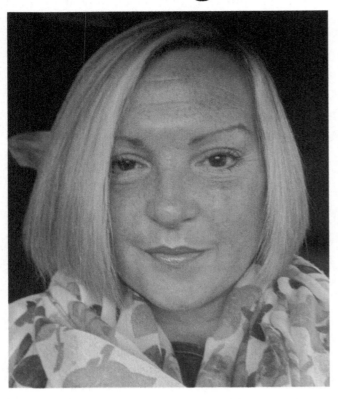

"Thankfully, I found a therapist who I instantly connected with and I've managed to sift through my life with Arthur and uncover Ruth...who happens to live with rheumatoid arthritis!"

My relationship with 'Arthur' has been a very long and tumultuous one. I was a healthy, sporty, fun loving 15 year old when I started experiencing swollen thumbs, knees and feet. Some days the pain was excruciating and I could hardly move, the next I was feeling nearly normal again, it was the most confusing time for me and my parents. A few months later I was diagnosed with RA at 16. We were actually relieved to finally know what was causing all this discomfort! The doctors were very positive and said it could all burn out as quickly as it arrived. We left thinking a simple anti-inflammatory would be the answer...How naive!

Within a few weeks it had affected every joint in my body and, at a time I was fostering my confidence and independence as a young woman, I became as reliant on my parents as I was the day I was born, unable to move, bathe, feed or toilet myself without their help. My world shrank to endless appointments with people in white coats, who seemed bemused at the speed of my deterioration. They threw every available drug at me, each one bringing the promise of relief but defiantly Arthur withstood them all. Four years later, aged 21, I had my first shoulder replaced. The subsequent years became a blurry cycle of surgery and recovery, a "whack a mole" like game, of "fixing" one joint and by then another needing attention. The most significant surgery was having my left knee replaced eight weeks before my wedding, enabling me to proudly walk down the aisle on my dad's arm towards Sean, the most incredible man who has loved and supported me for over 25 years. I believe the last count is around 50 surgeries to fuse and replace the worn out parts of me.

With the introduction of biologics and particularly tocilizumab, I began to feel that Arthur's grip was slowly loosening and finally the elusive "remission" was within my reach. To his credit, he had succeeded in his quest to leave a permanent trail of destruction in my body. But as the disease became less active my mind became far more active and I ever increasingly found myself reflecting on what I'd been through and more upsettingly what had been taken from me. Those years of self discovery had been stunted and overwhelmed with pain, immobility, a lack of independence and total dependence on others, for almost every aspect of my life.

I was married to an amazing man and became a stepmom to a then eight year old boy who I adore. Our wish was to extend our family with more children but unfortunately it just wasn't physically possible for me to care for a baby when I was barely able to care for myself. This was one of the many losses I found extremely difficult to come to terms with but in the midst of pain and operations I didn't have the energy to focus on it too much.

This past year, with the help of a wonderful

therapist I finally gave myself permission to grieve for the life I had wanted and hoped for, a life that wasn't dictated by Arthur, by pain and restrictions. I always tried to dismiss those thoughts and emotions. As they brought up negativity, guilt and shame, I would counteract them with positive thoughts like "Never mind, I am happy and grateful for the life I have" or, "I shouldn't feel sad that I don't have my own children, I have an amazing step son and three wonderful grandchildren"...which of course is all true! But deep down there was an emptiness, a wound that had never been given the chance to heal, I was ashamed to admit to myself and others that although 30 years had passed, I still didn't truly feel I had accepted my life with this illness. Slowly dissecting my past in therapy has enabled me to revisit some of the difficult times and offer myself kindness and compassion, being able to view my experience from a different perspective and with time passing, I have had the opportunity to grieve and find a level of acceptance I have always desired.

For many years I felt my identity as Ruth had been swallowed up by RA, I became a spectator of life and yearned to be a more active participant. Without having a career or being a mother, I struggled to find my purpose and it greatly impacted my self-worth and self-confidence. My mental health has at times been as arduous a journey as my physical health, with prolonged periods of severe depression accumulating in two "breakdowns." This triggered an abundance of shame and guilt, as I felt I had lost my composure and revealed the troubled girl behind the facade I had spent so long cultivating. The mask, I developed from years of self-imposed and external toxic positivity, had slipped. The pressure I felt to live up to the well-meaning, "You cope so well, you're so brave, you're always smiling" , had beaten me.

Thankfully, I found a therapist who I instantly connected with and I've managed to sift through my life with Arthur and uncover Ruth...who happens to live with rheumatoid arthritis! I have now begun to carve out a new and exciting path, I'm volunteering with two arthritis charities here in the UK which has renewed my sense of purpose. Creating a profile on Instagram, specifically for my life with RA, has been hugely positive too. There is a wonderfully supportive community of people online, all sharing their lived experiences. I have started writing poetry again which has been very therapeutic and I'm grateful to be able to share a couple here.

I am aware that one day Arthur may well be knocking on my door once more but with the love and support of my amazing husband, parents, friends, and family, I know I'll be just fine.

My Life with Arthur

Excuse me Mr Ritis...
Or can I call you Arthur?
I've some things to say to you,
Then you may leave thereafter.

Firstly, who do you think you are?
You really had no right
To interrupt my childhood
And steal it overnight.

Inside my adolescent body,
You raged a civil war.
My joints became your target;
Bone Crumbled more and more.

You high-jacked my identity,
my body, but not my spirit.
My parents taught me to be strong,
Positively we fought you with it.

You may not even recognize
The woman I've become
You took so much away from me
My chance to be a Mum

But with you now in remission
I'm accepting life this way
And I'm proud of where I am now
I'm a warrior with RA

So next time, my dear Arthur,
You decide to show your call,
I'll be waiting for your sorry arse
To grab you by the balls!

Coral Addison

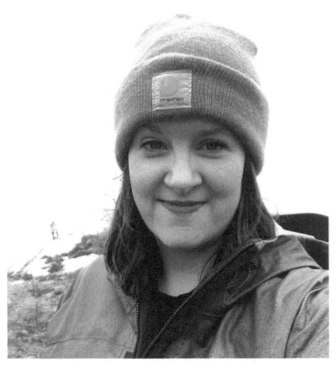

"I wish it was the end of my self doubt. The end of me wondering if I was just weak, lazy with a low pain threshold. These ideas never seem to go away though."

"The tests are all normal, I can see you again in six months if you would like?"

One of the many statements a doctor has made to me that caused me to doubt myself. Maybe it's not as bad as I think. Perhaps it is 'in my head' and I need to just stop thinking about it. It took me years to build up the courage to ask for help. I was referred to an internist who found nothing and referred me to a rheumatologist. I had waited months and driven two hours for this appointment.

Maybe it was in my head?

When the symptoms were mellow this was almost doable. However, some days they hit me like a freight train. I was blown off my feet by migratory joint aches and pains, along with crippling fatigue. I had a case of sciatica that never seemed to go away. Sometimes it was just a low growl, a gnawing pain in my lower back that radiated into my buttocks. At other times it was pulsing burning pain and I felt it around my groin and down the back of my leg. I couldn't sleep, I felt like I couldn't cope.

"You just need to do some strengthening and work on your posture," my rheumatologist told me. Cool. Perfect. Well actually I wanted to scream. Instead I just went numb. Tried to ignore the symptoms or mask them with hot baths, heating pads and working out.

Seven or eight years passed before I got up the courage to once again ask for help. I cried tears to my nurse practitioner. She actually listened and referred me back to the same rheumatologist. I had very, very low expectations at this point.

"Well I'll refer you to a physiotherapist for the sciatica. Sciatica is very common you know. I guess we can do a few SI joint x-rays as well." Meh, whatever. I give up.

A few weeks later I got a phone call. There was something different about this one. The doctors rushed, dismissive tone was off. She seemed more attentive. They had found indications of sacroiliitis and she wanted to send me for an MRI. I felt like the air was sucked out of the room. My mind spun. Part of me wanted to cry happy tears that it wasn't in my head. I wasn't just being whiny and weak. The other part of me was just shocked that anything had come up.

This was the beginning of my ankylosing spondylitis diagnosis. I wish it was the end of my self doubt. The end of me wondering if I was just weak, lazy with a low pain threshold. These ideas never seem to go away though. They pop back up and leave my mind spiraling. They make me doubt my own experiences and think that everyone around me thinks I'm faking it. Maybe one day I will be able to overcome this. But six months post diagnosis, and I still have a long way to go.

Kourtney Johnson

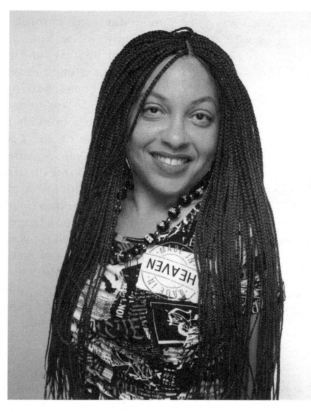

"You are stronger than you think."

I was 26 when I was diagnosed with RA. I thought it was an elders person's disease, only because my grandmother had it. I didn't know it ran in the family. Needless to say I was in shock. I thought my life was over. Now I have to watch my son to see if he will get it at 13. I'm 37 now and I've come to terms with it, but sometimes I do have my cry spells. I've had four knuckles replaced on my left hand because of my deformity and I'm going to end up getting my right one looked at also. I am still in recovery. I'm not able to bend my fingers just yet as it's a slow progress.

Has it taken a toll on me? Oh yes! Physically and mentally. So many nights I've cried, because of the pain I feel as I have RA throughout my body, from head to toe and from me being so tired. I can't have anymore kids, because of my RA and I'm still trying to process that. I have infusions every eight weeks. I'm doing physical therapy and occupational therapy four times a week. I have a therapist I see once a week. I've often questioned God asking why me?

Now I'm currently in school studying to become a clinical psychologist. I want to also specialize in rehabilitation counseling. While I was recovering from surgery I was still in school, to keep my mind off of reality. Reality that my left hand may or may not be like a normal person's hand. What is normal anyway? Even now, I have to worry about whether or not I'll have to see a spine doctor because of the issues I have with my neck. Did I mention I'm 37? People always ask me with everything I've been through, how am I still standing? My response is, God, my family and my medical team. They are my support system. I can't lie and say this journey has been a happy one. However, what I can say is it has made me stronger. I've pushed myself in ways I never thought were possible to me. I've also learned to listen to my body and slow down. Something I never do.

Jodie Humphries

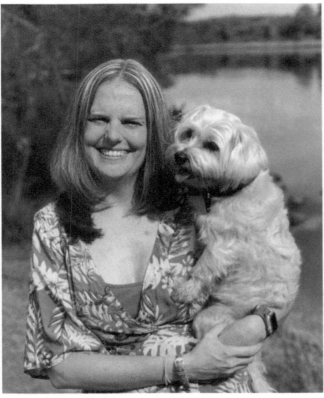

"Dealing with arthritis comes with a heavy emotional, mental and especially physical burden, dealing with medical professionals who have limited communication skills just adds to this burden. We as patients do need to work harder on advocating for ourselves, but this shouldn't be a burden shouldered only by the patients. Doctors need to have the skills to speak to and engage with their patients so that they don't avoid seeking help because they don't feel they'll be listened to or helped."

The Added Burden Of Dealing With Doctors Who Can't Communicate

There is a constant struggle when you've got a chronic illness between your old life, (before diagnosis), and your new one, (after diagnosis). But I think the biggest struggle for me was the journey to getting a diagnosis, which I am still struggling with.

Before even the thought of having any form of arthritis, I had been struggling to get doctors to understand my chronic fatigue. I haven't known the feeling of waking up refreshed since I was a teen. I'm now 37, and no doctor has ever really understood enough to search for a cause. So when my hands began hurting in 2021, I didn't really rush to the doctor to ask for answers. I had very little faith they could help. It wasn't until my hand pain kept me on the couch for a day, due to the pain, that I even considered going to the doctor.

It was a kind of surreal experience in that I went to the doctor, and they said, *"I think you have rheumatoid arthritis."* All before any blood tests or any knowledge of my family history. I was shocked. Here was a doctor who believed my symptoms and had a suggested diagnosis! My faith in the ability of doctors to help me was restored…for a very short time.

The blood tests came back, indicating I had RA. I found out half my dad's siblings had it and my symptoms matched the symptoms that usually come with early RA. But I needed a rheumatologist to confirm the diagnosis. I got the referral and headed off to the rheumatologist with this renewed faith in doctors. Unfortunately, that didn't last. My rheumatologist said he didn't believe it was RA, or he said it may be pre-clinical, which meant no course of treatment, just a, *"come back if things change."*

It was a hit I didn't expect. After the positive experience with the GP, I hoped to continue and get some solid assistance in managing this new diagnosis I thought I had. But it wasn't to be. I wasn't too upset because we were in the middle of a pandemic and an outbreak that led to a lock-down. So I was happy to not be on immunosuppressive drugs during this time, but I still felt like I was sent off to deal with this new situation on my own. I didn't even have another appointment booked, so I was sent off to sail along and see what would happen next with no real information.

Things changed when my life turned to chaos and this triggered what I thought was pre-clinical RA to turn clinical. My hands were inflamed and in pain to the point that I could not use them for two to three months over Christmas 2021. I had a telehealth appointment with my GP to get some anti-inflammatory painkillers and codeine. I'd had a day or two where I couldn't sleep due to the pain and wanted something on hand for those days. I also eventually booked another appointment with the rheumatologist but wasn't too confident I would walk away with any answers.

By the time I had the second appointment, my hands had calmed down and were pretty much back to normal. However, I had been in pain constantly for months, with inflammation going up and down at different times. I explained all of this to the rheumatologist and showed them photos of my hands when they were inflamed. He saw that there was a change but didn't want to start any treatment plan that I felt could help prevent the progression of the disease. I booked another appointment for a few months later and hoped things may change. I was given some prednisone to take during flares, but I felt my body was in a constant flare, so I stayed on it and still didn't see or feel any change.

When I eventually went back to the rheumatologist I explained that nothing had changed and I didn't see any difference when I was on the prednisone and when I was off it. I asked about methotrexate as a treatment option, which we'd discussed at the last appointment. I was given information about it to read.

A few things happened in this appointment that really frustrated me. The rheumatologist said they didn't want to put me on methotrexate because I am 37, unmarried, single and haven't had kids. I don't know if I will have kids, but to not be put on medication that could help my quality of life now because of a future possibility was infuriating. There was also this continued dismissal of my chronic pain because there was no inflammation the doctor could feel. I personally felt inflammation in my knee and saw some in my hands. Still, apparently, the doctor didn't, so it didn't exist.

The doctor also dropped a diagnosis I'd never heard before. I was under the impression I had the early stages of rheumatoid arthritis. Suddenly the rheumatologist said, *"Well, we decided last time that you have palindromic rheumatism."* I was so shocked. I had no idea what this was or when it had been decided. I didn't question anything in the appointment because I had moved, so getting a new rheumatologist was already on my mind. This just cemented it. I did some research when I left, and palindromic rheumatism can be a precursor to RA, but there is a distinct difference. The most significant difference is that the body returns to "normal" between flares with palindromic rheumatism. My understanding of this is that you have flares where you're in pain and have inflammation. Then in between these times, you feel no pain and have no inflammation. The body is meant to be completely symptom-free. This is where the supposed diagnosis of palindromic rheumatism confuses me for my circumstances. My body hasn't been "normal" or symptom-free for six months. I may not have constant inflammation, but I definitely have chronic pain, and my fatigue is worse than before I had any discussion of RA.

My fatigue was another bone of contention I had with the rheumatologist. I asked for ways to help with it. It was dismissed as part of my chronic fatigue. A few things here, I self-diagnosed my chronic fatigue because that's the only way to explain how I feel. Also, I wouldn't bring it up if it was my "usual" fatigue, I explained to the doctor that it was different, but it was still dismissed.

Being chronically ill is hard, emotionally, physically and mentally. Seeing doctors and having them dismiss your symptoms, making medical decisions based on future possibilities that are 100% your decision and not telling you the diagnosis, just add to the burden. I spent 20 years on and off trying to find an answer as to why I was chronically fatigued and got excited when I had an answer for my pain. Being dismissed or ignored about this new "diagnosis," (which I don't really have, I guess), has just put me back into a mental space where I don't have much faith in the medical profession. I will search for a new GP and rheumatologist in my new area, but it's frustrating that I feel like I have to start at the very beginning again.

I'm grateful for the online community I have found, not just of other RA warriors but other inflammatory arthritis and chronic illnesses. The online community gives me hope that I will find answers, get help and be able to manage this new illness in a way where I can live my life well.

Leigh Joiner

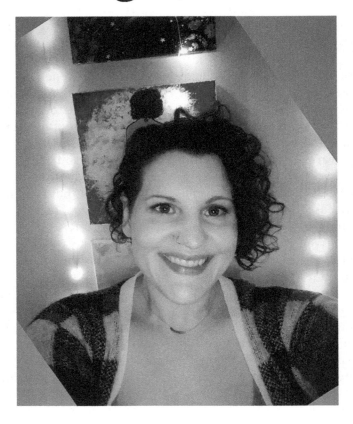

"I was confronted with the fact that I was once a vibrant, almost 30 year old now, to a, "you're too young to be sick," shell, limited to desk duty and canceled invites."

Like many, my arthritis story emerged like the perfect storm and I got caught in the eye of it. I started showing signs of inflammation/pain in the joints of my fingers. It was noticeable because I worked as a pharmacy technician. My specialty was oncology, preparing intravenous medications for our patients living with cancer and other hematological and chronic diseases. Dr visits were becoming more frequent and so were the antibiotics, steroids, pain meds, hand/finger splints, wraps, plus all the unsolicited advice.

I was confronted with the fact that I was once a vibrant, almost 30 yr old, to now a, "you're too young to be sick" shell, limited to desk duty and canceled invites. My identity, work role/status and job satisfaction, social presence and self esteem took a massive blow. I started on my first arthritis medication and when that one did not help, another one was added until I was taking over 10 medications a day and tried well over 20+ for various symptoms. At one point I was walking with a cane and approved for a handicap placard. My official diagnosis, after UCTD (undifferentiated connective tissue disease), was Sjogren's along with fibromyalgia.

My twin sister was diagnosed later that year with lupus and now has accompanying dx of Sjogren's. Also, my sister and I have EDS (ehlers danlos syndrome), hypermobility type III, because two chronic pain diseases were not enough! (insert dramatic eye roll). I have done a lot of detective work over the course of my disease and now know, trauma, environmental factors, STRESS, antibiotic overuse and much more were the catalyst for my disease progression.

I have never been one to give up without a fight and little did I know I would be fighting for more than just MY life. I was a volunteer/representative with the International Foundation for Autoimmune and Auto Inflammatory Arthritis (IFAA at the time), which allowed me to connect to others living with similar diseases. I was also provided opportunities to meet with others on a larger scale and advocate at the American College of Rheumatology Advocates for the arthritis conference in Washington, DC as well as participate in yearly fundraising with the Arthritis Foundation and Lupus Foundation. I have created lifelong connections with others from around the globe all because of arthritis... that one disease that people thought only older people could have.

My advocacy experiences and education, along with some encouraging coworkers and mentors, inspired me to continue my passion of working with others living with chronic diseases. I pursued my master's in clinical social work and currently hold my provisional license, exactly two hours away from being able to apply to sit for my national exam. One thing I did not account for was the fact that I am exactly where I need to be, working in the mental health field. Not surprisingly, many individuals who live with chronic diseases, such as autoimmune arthritis, live with chronic pain and are more likely to have poor mental health outcomes. I was lucky in that I received support from a therapist and I was in a graduate program that highlighted the importance of mental wellness, as well as being "shored up," as one of my favorite professors used to say, by some amazing humans. But there are so many that suffer; not provided with resources or the tools to help grieve or maneuver the chronic illness journey ahead.

I had reached non-medicated remission for a wonderful five years starting in 2016 and that came to a halt, with an accompanying additional diagnosis of ax-SpA (non-radiographic axial spondyloarthritis). That, however, will not stop me from advocacy or the purposeful work of helping others navigate this unpredictable terrain. Not only do I believe in remission, I believe in the other modalities and treatment options that continue to offer relief and hope for those of us who continue to fight every day to live a dynamic life.

Rachel Gehue

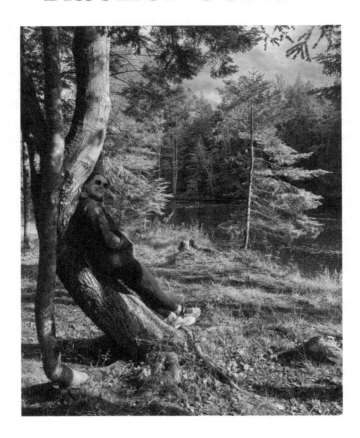

"I know now that it's okay to still be hurt over what this disease has taken from me and to mourn the life I thought I would have. But I've also learned to find joy in new places and to be grateful for things, in a way that I'm not sure I would've if I hadn't been diagnosed with arthritis. I mean, I'd still get rid of it in a second if I could, but in the meantime, I am grateful to everyone who has helped me build the life that I have, and I promise not to waste it."

When I turned 14, I was diagnosed with juvenile rheumatoid arthritis. There's a lot that goes on in the mind of a 14 year old to begin with. Your body is changing, you're trying to figure out the social constructs of junior high, and although you want to be yourself, you also want to fit in with everyone around you. You want attention, but only the right kind of attention. You don't really know who you are, but you also don't really know who you're not. It's confusing even at the best of times. I don't remember thinking about the future too much, but I guess I had my assumptions about what it would look like. That is, I never thought it would look very different. I know none of us have a clue when we're 14, but I really didn't have a clue.

I assumed that as I grew up, things in my life would evolve along with me, but I thought I would still be playing hockey, soccer, tennis and that I'd be ready for and able to do anything I wanted. I'd been heavily involved in sports since I was five. Why would that suddenly change? Why would I ever stop doing something I loved? It never really occurred to me that I wouldn't get a say in the matter. As my arthritis spread from head to toe, infecting every little nook and cranny of my skeleton, the list of things that I was physically capable of grew shorter and shorter. I began to feel more and more trapped in this body that I didn't recognize. Not only was I no longer able to do the high impact things like hockey, but then came the days where I couldn't even brush my own teeth. I was getting older – I should be getting more independent, not less. What kind of teenager needs help from her mom with basic hygiene?

I could go on and on about the abundance of physical issues I've experienced over the last decade: fusion surgeries, flares, injections, trips to the ER. That would be easy. What I've found most challenging to talk about has been the toll that something like arthritis, a predominantly physical disease, can have on your mental health. Learning to let go of the things that made me happy but that I was no longer able to do was one of the hardest things I've ever had to learn. In fact, 12 years later, I'm still learning how to do it. Your doctors prepare you for starting new medications and for the array of symptoms you may experience, but very rarely do they tell you that you may also have to prepare for an identity crisis as well. They don't tell you that there's a good chance, you'll be forced to be an entirely different person than who you thought you'd be and who you still feel like on the inside.

After I could no longer participate in the things I loved, I didn't really know what I was supposed to do. There was this intense disconnect between my mind and my body. I became afraid of trying anything new out of fear of suffering a bad flare. How was I going to find any sense of joy again? What would happen if I never did? Growing up with a body that wasn't doing what

it was supposed to was challenging enough, but then I found myself in a constant battle with my thoughts as well. Was I going to feel this lost forever? I didn't know if I'd be able to brush my own teeth in the morning, I certainly didn't know how I was going to build a life for myself.

The years after my diagnosis weren't entirely agonizing. I have wonderful, beautiful friends who have supported me in every way they could and we've made an abundance of amazing memories together. In fact, learning to be grateful for every little thing has been one of the few good things to come out of this diagnosis. I don't take anything for granted anymore. Over the years, I was able to go on trips with my family and out for drinks with my friends. I found a few new hobbies, like film photography and I was able to keep skiing most years. (I'm probably the only person in the world who appreciates the discomfort of rigid ski boots). On those weekends that I was able to get out of bed, I spent a lot of time trying to get out of my head too. Looking back now, with a more clear and mature perspective, I see that drinks with my friends quickly spiraled out of control because I let it. I couldn't be hurt by the things that I couldn't remember. My body was in such constant and severe agony, that oftentimes, the issues going on in my mind would get swept under the rug. I could only deal with so much at a time and my body took priority.

Over the years, I've learned how to shift those priorities and to take care of both my body and my mind. I'm not even close to having it all figured out, in fact, I still struggle a lot of the time. This disease is a beast that never seems to get tired, whereas I unfortunately get very tired, very easily. I know now that it's okay to still be hurt over what this disease has taken from me and to mourn the life I thought I would have. But I've also learned to find joy in new places that I'm not sure I would've if I hadn't been diagnosed with arthritis. I'd still get rid of it in a second if I could, but in the meantime, I am grateful to everyone who has helped me build the life that I have, and I promise not to waste it.

I'm on track to finally graduate from university this year. My timeline has been different than most, but I am capable of so much more than I thought I would be.

Edwin Mejia

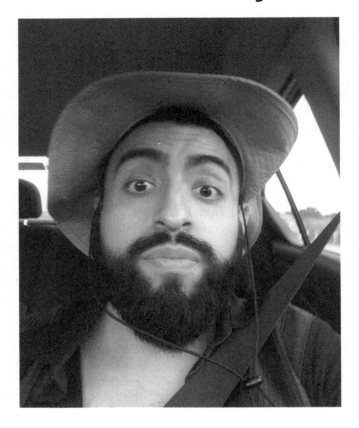

"This disease and all of its subsequent experiences have made me a more wholesome and loving individual. Or at least that's what I like to imagine."

I have battled rheumatoid arthritis for almost a decade now. I was diagnosed at age 23. I had to learn quickly how to balance my professional and personal life, while dealing with the obstacles that can come from RA. I have felt it all. Not just the chronic pain. But every emotion imaginable has claimed some form of residency in my head. It took me a while but my greatest achievement with this disease was to stop using it as my greatest weakness and transforming it into my greatest attribute. I went out and seeked adventure and fun.

I began to understand that a 10 day vacation may include me laying in bed for a day or two, to either recover from an exhausting adventure or fighting a flare-up. And that was fine. Fine because I had grown up mostly as a homebody. An introvert. But I have always had a constant fascination with travel. So instead of using this disease as an excuse to deny the request to "go out," I used it to transform myself into a mix of all the travel channel hosts from the late 2000s. And through those travels I found a new way of connecting with people. Turns out walking with a noticeable limp is the ultimate ice breaker. This disease and all of its subsequent experiences have made me a more wholesome and loving individual. Or least that's what I like to imagine.

Vanessa Ferrante

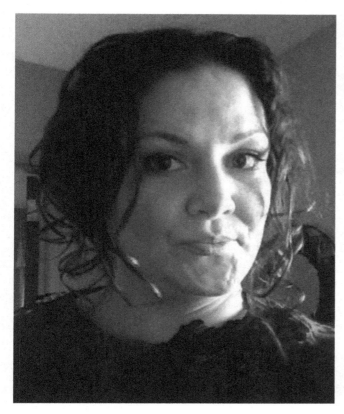

"Don't give up! I say that A LOT! Even on my darkest days, I like to remind myself that I'll get through every doctor visit, injection, flare, and conversation about me and it's because I am strong and a warrior and I have the most amazing people in my life! I couldn't be more blessed!"

As I sit here writing this, I am missing out on my best friend's milestone birthday party because I have been suffering from the worst PsA flare I've ever experienced. I'm feeling all of the feelings, depression, anxiety, fatigue, heartache, but most importantly, disappointment. I am a natural-born people pleaser, so when I can't be there for someone I love because my PsA gets in the way, it sends me to a dark place.

I was diagnosed with PsA almost four years ago but no matter how many years you've been suffering with this, it never gets easier. While my friends and family don't know what it's like to experience the flares from PsA, they are always supportive and understanding when I have to cancel an event that has been booked days/weeks/months in advance. I couldn't be more blessed/grateful to have such a loving group of 'framily' in my life. PsA isn't easy but finding communities and having a badass team who supports you, even on your darkest days, really does make all the difference in the world for your mental health.

I have people ask me all the time, *"How are you feeling? Are you healthy? Are you doing ok? Can I do anything for you?"* and to be honest, hearing those questions used to trigger my anxiety and sometimes it still does. I'm like a deer in headlights! I would start sweating and overthinking, trying to figure out the best lie to tell that person so they would think I'm ok. My responses would be short and sweet: *"Sure, I'm doing great! Everything is wonderful, thank you for asking! Haven't felt better! I'm alive so that's all that matters,"* all whilst smiling and sinking deeper and deeper into that dark depression because I didn't wanna burden anyone with a truthful answer. I'm learning to let go of what I can't control (I'm a Gemini so it's hard) and when someone asks me those questions, I know they are asking because they genuinely care about me and my health. So they deserve a truthful answer whether it be bad or good, even though I do hope for more good days to report to than bad!

Don't give up! I say that A LOT! Even on my darkest days, I like to remind myself that I'll get through every doctor visit, injection, flare, and conversation about me and it's because I am strong and a warrior and I have the most amazing people in my life! I couldn't be more blessed!

Steff Di Pardo

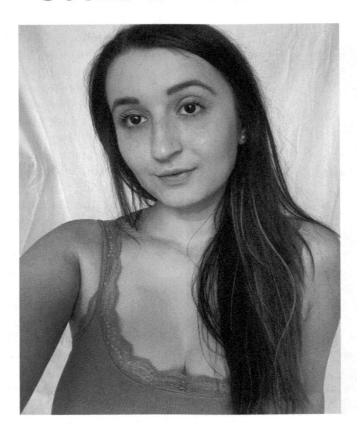

"Over the years, I've had many ups and downs when it comes to my mental health with this disease. It really eats at you some days. Others, I can accept that this is my life and it will be forever."

I've had arthritis for over five years now. I developed it at the age of 21 and I can't tell you how much that affected my mental health in my early twenties. Actually, I can tell you. And I will.

It was incredibly isolating to experience something like arthritis at such a young, crucial part of my life. I went from a healthy, newly 21 year old to a bedridden 21 year old in a matter of days. It was terrifying and I had no idea of what was going on in my body.

Pretty obviously, my mental health declined over the months that I was bedridden. I barely talked to my friends because I didn't know how to explain what was going on. I had no idea this was arthritis and it was so hard to explain.

"No, I wasn't coming back to work yet. No, I don't know what's wrong. I'm just in pain all the time, but no one knows why."

I started to isolate myself from my co-workers and friends. I was tired of telling them that I didn't know what was going on. As confusing as it was for them, it was 10 times more confusing for me. I was seeing my doctor every other week at this point, with no real answers. Just referrals to specialists.

Specialist appointments in Canada can take months to even years to get. I was referred to a neurologist and a rheumatologist to see what was going on. Over these months of waiting, the anxiety just got worse and worse.

I saw the neurologist first, and he had no idea what was going on. It didn't have anything to do with neurology. That appointment was disappointing. I remember being so upset that he didn't have any answers for me. The wait for answers with anxiety just takes so much out of you.

I wanted to go back to my normal, 21 year old life! Little did I know, that life was never coming back.

The anxiety got worse and worse as I awaited my rheumatologist appointment. Six months after the referral, I finally saw him. He suspected something right away and sent me for further testing.

I finally felt heard and seen! Things were going somewhere after this appointment! In my head, I still thought this could be a quick fix and I could go on with my life. Four months later, I found out that wasn't the case.

I was diagnosed with ankylosing spondylitis at age 22. I never thought I would get arthritis at such a young age but that was my ignorant thinking. I didn't know it was possible.

Over the years, I've had many ups and downs when it comes to my mental health with this disease. It really eats at you some days. Others, I can accept that this is my life and it will be forever.

It's when the flare-ups happen that I tend to have a harder time dealing with my mental health. When I flare up, I tend to retreat to the ways I did when I was 21. I isolate myself and become upset. It's not an easy disease to deal with! Being unable to get out of bed on my own sometimes can be very frustrating and strips me of my independence.

Depression really sinks in with arthritis sometimes. I see other people my age, (now 26), going out and partying without a thought in their mind of whether they can move tomorrow or not. I have to think about that every single time I leave the house to do something. Even if I have a glass of wine at home, I may not be able to move the next day!

I'm lucky that I have a good support system. Once diagnosed, I turned to Instagram to find support. I found an entire community of chronically ill people that uplift each other and are always there for me. It's helped the depression and anxiety of this illness so much. I know there's always someone there for me to relate to me, even if they don't have the same illnesses as me!

My mental health is still impacted every single day with arthritis. I've just found better ways to cope and find support from my community. That helps an immense amount.

Laura Jean

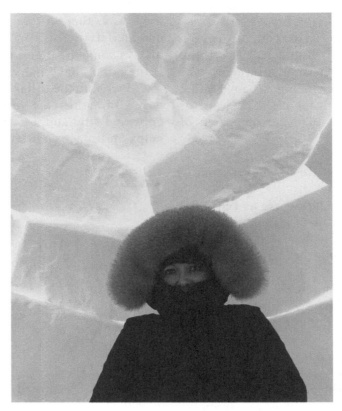

"Chronic illness has taken my life on a detour I wasn't expecting, but it's still a beautiful ride!"

I will never forget the day I was diagnosed with rheumatoid arthritis. It was like a sucker punch to the gut. The words felt heavy in the air, yet were strangely accompanied by a light sense of relief to finally, after six years of pain and struggles, have an answer, to know what exactly I was up against.

With nothing to equip me, except a piece of paper with a new prescription jotted on it, a single sheet of information about the drug and possible side effects....there I was...walking out of the hospital... left to figure it out on my own. My mind was racing. It was a lot to take in. It took time to process it all.

My life was forever changed from that moment and I was only just beginning to see how it would affect every aspect of my life.

There were goals I had that I knew I may realistically never be able to achieve, or at the very least not in the timeline that I hoped to achieve them. My focus needed to shift to finding a way to feel better and to function in day-to-day life. At this point, just feeding myself with a fork, or cutting the food on my plate with a knife, was a mountain-like challenge. So reaching for goals beyond that didn't seem appropriate.

After a brief period of grieving, (*grieving a chronic illness diagnosis is very similar to grieving the loss of a loved one...because there certainly is a loss: the loss of the life you had expected for yourself*), I managed to accept my new diagnosis.

I have rheumatoid arthritis. I have rheumatoid arthritis. I HAVE rheumatoid arthritis. It took some practice before the words would roll off my tongue. And if I'm being completely honest, it took a few times of relying on spell check before I could even write it out.

Once I accepted the diagnosis, I experienced an intentional mindset shift.

I have rheumatoid arthritis BUT rheumatoid arthritis will not have me.

RA may attack my body but I still control my thoughts and my reactions and I am determined to not let it get the best of me. My diagnosis is an opportunity. Granted, not one that I would choose, if I had the choice, but it is an opportunity nonetheless. It is an opportunity for me to grow, for me to dig deep, for me to learn, to problem solve, and to inspire others.

I will not be a victim of RA, I will be an RA conqueror!

With that mindset, I started my quest. My quest to conquer RA...or to go down trying. I first had to educate myself about the disease. The doctor had simply told me it was an autoimmune condition with chronic inflammation, but it was time I learned the nitty-gritty details of RA so that I knew what I was up against.

Next, I connected with others who had RA. When I was first diagnosed I didn't know a single person who had RA. I started to talk about it with family and friends and they would refer to friends they had, who also had RA and would put us in touch with each other, so we could chat and I could ask questions. I also searched online for people with RA who were sharing their story. I found online communities and organizations who offer information and support for people with various forms of arthritis.

The next phase of my quest was climbing from the "backseat" into the "driver's seat" for my healing journey. It was time I took action and made changes in my life to support my health goals.

I started to invest in my health and make it a priority in my day-to-day life. I made adjustments in my work schedule to scale back the physical demands on my body. I made drastic changes to my diet, so that food was a fuel for my body instead of something that bogged it down. I made appointments with naturopaths, massage therapists, and acupuncturists...even when it was financially challenging and I had to sell items around the house, just to be able to afford the appointment. My health was worth more than the clutter around our home and I became determined to invest in it.

My quest continued with finding solutions for the daily challenges I was experiencing. I've always loved brainstorming ideas and thinking outside the box, so each struggle that I faced in the day I viewed as a puzzle that needed solving. What solution could I come up with to make this task easier and less painful?

The solutions would sometimes come in the middle of the night when I would lay awake. At other times, the solutions appeared as I did extensive research online. Either way, I felt a small victory every time I managed to make a task easier or less painful.

After several "victories" and noticing improvements in my life from the changes I was making, plus the life hacks I was implementing, I wanted to do more to conquer RA. I wanted to help others do the same. I wanted to be able to share my experience, in the hopes of it helping others to have their own victories.

So, unexpectedly, I began an entirely new online quest of sharing my story. At first it was just through Instagram, where I shared the tips and tricks that were making a difference in my life. When that was well received and I was receiving frequent messages from other RA warriors who said that my tips were helping them and bringing relief and hope. My quest expanded to include operating a blog, where I can dive deep into all things rheumatoid arthritis and the simple solutions that can make a big difference in managing life with it.

Learning how to set up, design and operate a blog was something I never thought I could do but if RA has taught me anything, it's that I can do hard things! So I took on the challenge, and like other challenges, or opportunities in my life, I just found a way to make it work.

Remembering back to how I felt that first day when I walked out of the hospital with a diagnosis and little else to equip me for life with RA, it brings me such joy to know I have now created resources to help others with a diagnosis of rheumatoid arthritis, to not feel alone and to have some tools to help them cope and manage their new life.

My RA isn't (yet) in remission, but with the physical and mental improvements that I have experienced since that day of diagnosis, I DO feel like an RA conqueror.

Chronic illness has taken my life on a detour I wasn't expecting, but it's still a beautiful ride!

Daisy Gallardo

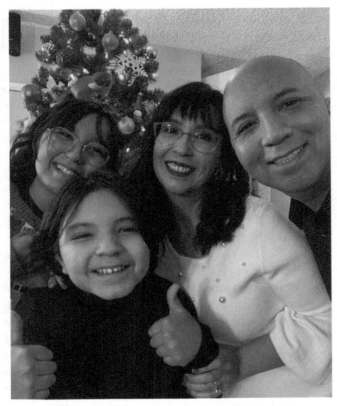

"Although arthritis is partly an enemy in my life and honestly very difficult, learning to accept its perils with its gifts has been a life changing opportunity."

I'm a month away from my 39th birthday. When I look back on my arthritis journey, it's hard to believe all the major challenges I've endured and all I continue to survive. So much has changed in just a few years. Although my arthritis symptoms began at the age of 14, it took me decades to finally get a diagnosis. I recall the sudden flare ups and progression of duration and severity of pain throughout my 20s.

By then, I had obtained medical insurance through my husband and never thought I would have been ignored for the majority of my doctor visits. I suffered pelvic, hip, and lower back pain through both of my pregnancies and doctors would blame it on lifting incorrectly, sleeping in an awkward position, anxiety, depression, and some just thought I was exaggerating. After dozens of ER visits, many doctor visits, physical therapy, pain meds and what felt like a giant waste of time, I decided to stop reaching out to doctors whenever I'd flare up.

I was a kindergarten teacher and I had adjusted to the idea that at least once a year my back would eventually give out and I'd call out of work. These intense pelvic and back flare ups were so painful, I could barely walk and after a week in bed, I somehow recovered. This would happen at least twice a year and sometimes lasted up to two weeks. Instead of relying on doctors, I found some pain relief through acupuncture.

One summer, I started to develop a panic disorder as I would have panic attacks often. I was overwhelmed by the pressure of being a mom, teacher, my unexplained debilitating pain, medical gaslighting, and toxic familial relationships. The panic attacks were terrifying and my body couldn't keep up either. Mentally, I was very drained and felt so lost. I started to take long walks around my neighborhood, until one day I started to limp halfway through the walk. Then, it was as if that caused a domino effect in my body. Soon my hands started hurting, shoulders, ankles, etc. I dreaded going back to the doctor but I had to. I was referred to a rheumatologist who was a huge disappointment. He appeared bothered by my presence and told me to revisit when my hands were extremely swollen.

About a month later, I developed what I thought were fainting spells, but now know this as extreme fatigue. I saw a neurologist to treat these symptoms and was diagnosed with migraines and given depression medication. The very next day, I suddenly couldn't get up from the couch and walk. My life has never been the same again. I thought I could sleep it off, but much to my surprise, my legs felt like heavy weights in the morning and my husband rushed me to the hospital. There they performed a spinal tap and many other tests and since I had seen the neurologist the day before, they attributed all symptoms to migraines. I was floored. There I was in a wheelchair because of migraines? I knew this wasn't why, so I begged my doctor to run more tests.

Because the rheumatologist I'd seen two months prior thought nothing of my joint pain, my primary doctor blamed everything on my unwillingness to walk. She didn't want me to seek a second opinion with another rheumatologist. She told me to stop wasting insurance money on more testing. I continued to see the neurologist and was prescribed higher doses of antidepressants.

Meanwhile, I was trying my hardest to work for a new school as a teacher while learning how to manage my new life in a wheelchair. Seven months later, I decided to change insurance plans to a Preferred Provider Organization (PPO) in order to get to the bottom of my disability. I soon made the switch and scheduled a pain management visit. They handed me a pain questionnaire in which I was instructed to mark an x where I felt pain on the drawing of a female body. I pretty much marked up the whole page and when I consulted with the doctor, he told me this wasn't normal and referred me to a rheumatologist. I was relieved to visit a new rheumatologist who diagnosed me in just two weeks. She said I had advanced psoriatic arthritis and fibromyalgia. I couldn't believe that so many doctors had missed it! She even read an old pelvic mri, which already indicated pelvic erosions, scar tissue, and inflammation. I also had small erosions in my fingers and wrists. She briefly discussed biologic treatments and gave me hope that I'd be able to walk again soon. I thought this was it, my life would go back to how it was… boy was I so wrong.

After failing numerous treatments very quickly, she referred me to a new rheumatologist. I felt defeated because each time I started a new treatment, I'd respond well and was able to go to work without a wheelchair for two to three days, then all of the sudden, I'd collapse midday, leaving me confused and ashamed. A few years later, I discovered I had spinal and hip deformities contributing to more pain and had surgeries to correct the problems in 2019.

The physical aspect of this journey is much too long so I'll update you on my current status seven years later:

- My current and amazing rheumatologist has realized my body fights off all treatments after a few months, making this disease extremely difficult to treat.

- I'm only able to walk for about 20 minutes and I must rest in between tasks.
- I use a cane and scooter for longer outings or during a bad flare up.
- I'm now about to start on my 10th biological in seven years.
- Thanks to unknowingly completing the required years of teaching to obtain disability benefits and my severe disability, I was able to qualify for disability benefits after almost one year.

This disease has changed every aspect of my life. Although this may sound outrageous, it has given me the most important gift in my life, self love and self advocacy. It forced me to reevaluate the things in my life that were causing chaos and pain. It has also forced me to face the emotions and trauma I had put at the back of my mind for so long. I realized just how much emotional pain and suffering I was carrying. I began taking accountability for not putting my needs above everyone else's. It made me aware of my uncharted empowerment as a woman in this world. I've become aware that my initial feelings of shame toward my disability and not being able to work, were my internal ableism. I'm learning to value my worth for the person I am, not what I'm not able to do. Chronic pain has changed me, but not completely for the worst.

Sometimes it feels unrelenting and suffocating, but I'm learning how to navigate living the best life I can. Thanks to my circumstances, I have let go of abusive relationships, started therapy, and even begun taking my passion of singing more seriously.

These are things I'm sure I would have continued to ignore had it not been for this illness that has brought me to my knees. I'm a survivor and I will never give up. I hope to be able to stabilize my disease enough to someday work as a part-time substitute teacher and until then, I will continue to nourish my body and soul and honor myself every step of the way.

My husband and children have been part of my determination to search for my inner peace and healing. Although arthritis is partly an enemy in my life and honestly very difficult, learning to accept its perils with its gifts has been a life changing opportunity.

Puisy Luong

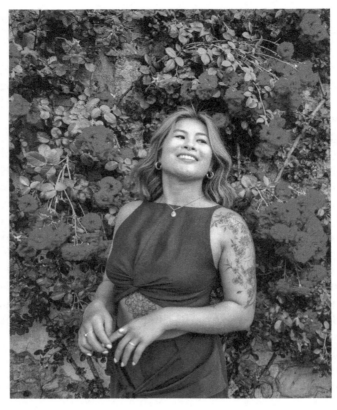

"One of my biggest pet peeves is when you first tell someone about your condition and they respond with "Oh my grandma has that." RA is not just an "old person" disease. I'm openly discussing it in the hope of not only having more control and acceptance of the situation, but to support other young people in feeling less lonely in their struggles."

I'm 31 years old and I want to share my story. October 2012, around the age of 21, I noticed a dull ache in my feet after a night out and some rock climbing. I didn't think too much of it but the ache persisted despite some time. Naturally concerned, I decided to see my GP.

They asked whether I had an accident, along with some other questions which were all inconclusive. After multiple x-rays, scans, blood tests and a podiatrist referral, it was then determined that I had early rheumatoid arthritis. By this point it was March 2013 and I was 22 years old. Due to my age, arthritis was not the first diagnosis. The initial years started off manageable. I was taking hydroxychloroquine which kept the symptoms at bay.

I noticed the pain returning in 2017. The consistent ache in my feet throughout the day, struggling to walk up and down the stairs, wrist pains, etc. Hydroxychloroquine alone was not enough to tackle my worsening symptoms. I started sulfasalazine alongside my existing medications.

My symptoms stabilized leading up to October 2020 and my doctor recommended that I completely stop the hydroxychloroquine. There were several factors that I suspected, stress, age, the pandemic but suddenly I felt more pain than I've ever experienced. There's no way for me to be sure but I'm certain dropping the hydroxychloroquine and stress were some of the key factors of my relapse.

To my relief, I was made redundant in December 2020. I welcomed the break in work. I spent Nov/Dec 2020 hoping the pain would pass. Jan/Feb 2021 I struggled to sleep with my symptoms keeping me up at night. I started feeling pain in new parts of my body. The disease eventually progressed to my hands, meaning that I could no longer form a fist. Today I have joint deformities in my right hand. Lol, I call it my witchy hand.

In true British fashion, the constant rain was torture on my body. I got some brief relief during summer when London was blessed with some sun (lol finally). Eventually I found some days I could no longer match the walking pace of my friends/family and my RA was much more "visible" than before. It really challenged my identity as a young woman.

October 2021, my doctor agreed sulfasalazine was not effective and I've since been on a course of steroids and prescribed methotrexate. The steroids helped as a short term, immediate relief to the pain and inflammation of my joints. I'm responding well to the methotrexate and having monthly blood tests for monitoring.

Since my relapse and flair, one of my major battles has been with anxiety. I haven't physically and mentally been the same since 2020. I now find myself worrying about things which I previously did not consider.

My first love is bachata. I'm conscious of how I'm perceived outwardly, especially as a dancer. Bachata is a beautiful and sensual partner dance that requires flexibility and core strength. I'm cautious of who I dance with nowadays, finding myself often saying no if an overzealous lead asks for a dance. It almost feels like a taboo to decline a dance in the world of bachata and I can't help but feel guilty for explaining myself each time. Having an "invisible" illness, I find myself in a constant state of identity crisis, hidden under this perceived veil of "health."

This year is the first time I've been able to travel since the pandemic. I'm grateful to travel with friends and resume adventures this year but I'm also conscious of my body's new "pace." Where I was able to keep up, nowadays I struggle. I'm coming to terms with it slowly and learning to embrace my own rhythm in life.

I'm also a wannabe aerialist. During class, my instructor asked if the silks caused any pain to my hands. Lol, well, I responded with, *"I'm always in pain."* It was a bit of a trick question, but he understood my response as someone who also suffers from chronic pain. Due to my stubborn personality I've never really been one to give up on things. But after developing arthritis in my hands which weakened my grip and damaged my joints, I felt so dejected and hopeless that I seriously considered quitting. But I'm glad I didn't. Fast forward to a year later, I'm responding well to methotrexate and still going strong with the silks.

Part of gaining control of your narrative is having acceptance. Something I wanted to do this year was to speak more openly about chronic illness. Perhaps even greater than the physical struggles, are the mental struggles that come with RA. The feeling of your body betraying you, low body image, which then contributes to the challenges of dating with a chronic illness, medication anxiety, social isolation etc.

One of my biggest pet peeves is when you first tell someone about your condition, and they respond with, *"Oh my grandma has that."* RA is not just an "old person" disease. I'm openly discussing it in the hope of not only having more control and acceptance of the situation, but to support other young people in feeling less lonely in their struggles. I had a conversation with a friend recently and being more vocal has shown me that there are so many young people living with chronic illnesses, unbeknownst to you. Talking to someone you trust is the first step towards feeling less lonely and building a support system.

Somewhere out there is also another tatted-up baddie with RA, multiple ear piercings, who loves life despite its challenges. RA is complete pants but I'm learning to live more presently and slowly because of it. I've gained appreciation for the smaller beauties in life, continuously learning about myself and how to manage my physical, spiritual, and mental health.

I just wanted to say, it's OK, this card would have never been dealt if you couldn't handle it. I want to highlight the realities of RA but also show that your life doesn't need to stop with chronic illness. You can still experience beauty in life, maybe just a little slower than others. Your body is meant to move at a pace in which it allows, listen to her. RA is part of your life, accept it, but it doesn't define you. You're doing your best.

Kerry Wong

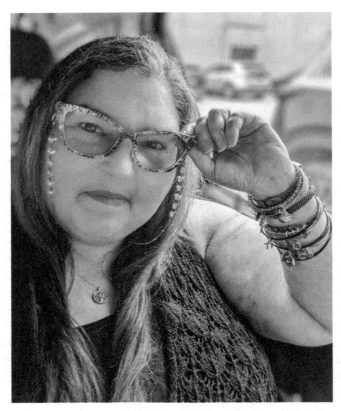

"Having arthritis makes me feel like I'm living with the seven dwarfs."

Am I Snow White?

It seems like a silly question. I mean, I am pretty fair-skinned and I did have a stepmother, but she never tried to have me killed. I don't come from royalty, I'm not the fairest in the land and I absolutely don't love housework. That said, I feel like her in one significant way: *Having arthritis makes me feel like I'm living with the seven dwarfs.*

You know the cast: Dopey, Happy, Grumpy, Bashful, Sleepy, Sneezy, and Doc. They whistle while they work, and care for Snow White when she's hiding from the wicked queen. What you may not know is all the arthritis.

While the word arthritis literally means inflammation of the joint(s), the term actually refers to over 100 conditions and joint inflammation is only one of many symptoms. They can affect any organ and can even cause systemic (full-body) symptoms as well.

In my left hip, I've got what most people think of: osteoarthritis, a degenerative condition caused by wear and tear of the joint, often from age, weight, or overuse. Bursitis and tendinitis make that one hip even more painful and I'll probably need to have it replaced in the not-too-distant future. I also have a number of autoimmune and inflammatory conditions including rheumatoid arthritis, sarcoidosis, and sjögren's syndrome, which affect the entire body, including the joints. Finally, I have fibromyalgia, which falls under the arthritis umbrella as well and brings with it a wide variety of symptoms.

All of these conditions have a profound effect on me and not only physically. They have limited my ability to do so many things, from walking around the block to working around the clock. They have a mental and emotional impact too, both from the conditions themselves and from the limitations they lead to.

Ultimately, these conditions leave me feeling like I'm living with Snow White's friends, and they're really rubbing off on me.

I feel Dopey.

There's one symptom we don't talk about much because it can be especially difficult to talk about while we're experiencing it: brain fog. When this hits, it can be difficult to put a sentence together. I can re-read a paragraph or rewind a TV show multiple times and still have no idea what it was about. On the way home from my infusion treatment one day, I actually asked my mom, *"Was I just about to say something else, or did I already say something else?"* It can definitely make me feel dopey.

I feel Happy.

While I would not wish arthritis of any kind on anyone, there is definitely one wonderful thing that comes with this disease: the arthritis community. When I meet other people living with arthritis (either in person or virtually), there is an instant connection. I have found people who truly understand what I'm going through when the rest of the world does not. I have an incredible source of support, laughter, ideas, and information in my arthritis family. That certainly makes me happy.

I feel Grumpy.

There are infinite reasons to be upset with arthritis and though I am generally a positive, cheerful, optimistic person, even I get depressed, anxious, and downright grumpy at times. It can take a while to find the right doctors and some of the wrong ones can be infuriating. I've had doctors who were dismissive of my experience, my knowledge, and my wishes. When they couldn't figure out what was wrong or how to treat it, they said it was "just depression" and left me at that. Living in constant pain and not getting answers or relief can be especially frustrating. When others around don't understand, it can impact jobs and relationships, too. These can easily make me grumpy.

I feel Bashful.

Bashful is probably one of the last words most people would use to describe me. I am not shy about sharing my story or speaking up for what's right through a variety of media. But when I am flaring (a period of amplified symptoms, more severe than usual), I generally retreat into myself. I don't have the mental energy, or the desire, to reach out to anyone , or respond to any messages. I might scroll through a few social media posts but I don't post anything anywhere. I surely seem bashful.

I feel Sleepy.

There is a level of fatigue that comes with arthritis that is completely unfathomable for anyone without it. The tiredness is so strong that I can barely keep my eyes open but it is not relieved by any sleep. I can't even fall asleep, or I wake from it frequently. There's even a word we use, "painsomnia," for when we develop insomnia because of the pain. That fatigue envelops my entire body, so picking up my phone requires more energy than I can exert. Moving, writing, talking, thinking … all of these become too much effort for me. I feel lethargic, beyond sleepy.

I feel Sneezy.

This is probably the easiest to relate. Because many of my arthritis conditions stem from the immune system, both they and the treatments for them leave me immunocompromised. That means I'm literally always sick. The systemic inflammation can lead to symptoms like fevers, chills, and yes, even sneezes! I take 27 pills per day, and I have an injection and an infusion every week, not to mention pain medications and non-medical treatments that I use as needed. Sneezy is only the beginning.

I feel (like a) Doc.

Like far too many in the arthritis community, it took years for me to get an accurate diagnosis. I spent four years with doctors turning me away because I didn't look sick and another four years with rotating misdiagnoses as they tried to figure out what was wrong. I had to do my own research on symptoms, diagnoses and treatments. I had to push for my doctors to perform diagnostic tests I'd learned about and to try certain medications I'd read about. One specialist was so impressed with my knowledge, he asked if I worked in the medical field. *"Yes,"* I said. *"I'm a professional patient."* Like a doc.

It's taken a long time to come to terms with this enchanted life, with everything (and everyone) that comes along with arthritis. But what it's taught me, to quote Snow White herself, is that *"I'm sure I'll get along somehow. Everything's going to be alright."* And even with arthritis, I can have my happily ever after.

Kelly Conway

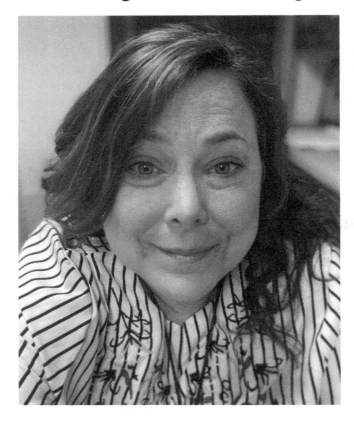

"Connecting with fellow patients can help form a sense of community when living with chronic illness. For me finding strangers who understood what it was like to live in chronic pain was a revelation."

It's a Stranger Thing

My diagnosis journey was a roller coaster. I was originally diagnosed with Sjogren's syndrome and told by a rheumatologist, *"At some point, you'll develop rheumatoid arthritis or lupus."* Foreboding, right? I was never diagnosed with Lupus but I have had a revolving door of diagnoses. I've been diagnosed with RA, psoriatic arthritis, ankylosing spondylitis, and spondyloarthropathy. Although my symptoms never changed, my diagnosis changed to help me access medications to relieve my symptoms. Some treatments gave me relief from debilitating pain and swelling, while others allowed me to feel the burning hell that is autoimmune arthritis.

Through it all, people in my life ask, *"What is wrong with you?"* Honestly, it is confusing enough for me to have revolving diagnoses, I can only imagine how my friends and family felt. Soon, I found it difficult to talk about my diseases to people who cared about me. I found myself never saying that I felt good because the next time I felt terrible those people freaked out. I remember my aunt practically yelling at me, *"What did you stop doing? You felt great the last time we talked."* It soon became easier to write about my feelings and experiences on social media than to confide in those closest to me. It may sound absurd, but strangers helped me learn how to live better with chronic illness.

I found people on the Internet understood me better than many life-long friends and even family. Living with chronic illness, I struggle daily to get through the simplest of tasks because of chronic pain. My family and friends are very supportive and I know I am lucky, but even when they try to understand my pain, they often don't get it. This is especially true when dealing with medication. My dear friend excitedly called me one day to see if I saw the ad for a new medication that helped people like me. Sadly, that medication was one of the first I tried and it didn't help me at all. I felt like a failure for not responding positively to a drug that helps millions according to the TV ads! According to TV on some meds, I should be able to ride my bike, play frisbee with my dog, and work in my garden. My reality when medication is working is being able to fasten buttons, shower, and reach for items on the top shelf of the grocery store. I call a day like that a win. Overtime, I felt like a stranger not only in my body, but within my circle of friends and family.

Living with a chronic illness is very difficult and it can lead to depression. If I need to vent about the difficult times, I find people close to me either pity me or try to fix things for me. Then there are the people who just want to cure me with all kinds of diets and treatments. Sometimes, I just need someone to listen and not judge. A therapist has helped a lot in terms of dealing with depression and learning to cope, but social media has also played an important role in chronic illness journey.

Finding people on social media who understood when I posted about living in pain was a revelation. I can post how hard it is to vacuum because my hand keeps going numb and I'll get Sally Smith from Any-town, USA responding to me with, *"Me too!"* or *"I get it!."* Some people even offer advice that really works. The simple fact of knowing I am not the only one going through these issues is reassuring. I don't share everything online, but I share enough to gain perspective and support when I need it.

Finding fellow chronic illness warriors helped decrease my feelings of isolation and depression. Through social media, I was able to find a community to get me through the tough spots. Over the years, I've learned how to communicate more effectively with my friends and family regarding my disease, but I still cherish those online who provided me a sense of community when I needed it most. They have helped me learn that living with multiple chronic illnesses isn't the end of the world, rather it is just another way of living in the world and it is often wonderful.

Andrea Dunn

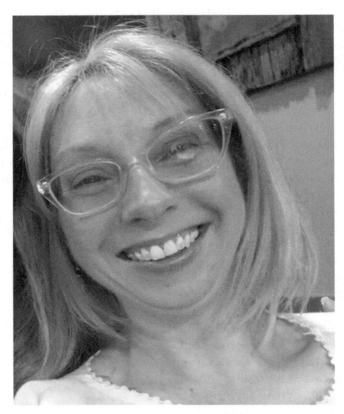

"Two years went by. I lost my confidence in knowing my body. I lost trust in medical professionals. My head was spinning and I felt defeated."

This story starts when I was about 34 years old. At this point I had been diagnosed with JRA for 11 years and probably had it for 10 more. My professional trade is in sports medicine, I am an athlete trainer. This is kind of ironic - a way I know God is humorous because I was basically a muscle and joint specialist and I had a joint disease. I was having terrible hip pain. It had increased over the years to be debilitating. I knew it was time for me to seek a professional. My rheumatologist had suggested a hip surgeon that he trusted. Because of my great interaction with him I decided to also trust the surgeon and see what he could do for me. I had already exhausted all of my ideas as an athletic trainer and it was time to go to the next level. I had to accept that I had no idea what this kind of pain meant. It was new and not like anything I learned about in college that my patients would feel.

I was looking forward to this conversation with the surgeon because I imagined him holding me to a higher standard, since my expertise was in a similar field. I was certain my use of medical terms to a superb degree would help me bypass some of the pomp and circumstance that often goes with the first consult of injury evaluation. You know, the speech given that you just need to rest it for two weeks, take advil, ice and elevate and then come back in a month to see how it's doing.

When I arrived the nurse sent me to get x-rays. I was relieved and also excited because I was prepared like a good little patient. I had brought my previous x-rays from 12 years ago so he could compare. Why did I have x-rays in college? Let me tell you about the previous history to that left hip...as it all ties together.

When I was away at college, 21 years old, I got into a really bad car wreck when I fell asleep at the wheel. When the rescue squad came to save me and rip open my door with the "jaws of life," they inadvertently took my left leg with them and broke my femur (the largest bone in the body.) I was rushed to a local North Carolina hospital and then air vacced to an even bigger hospital. A week later and I was out with a metal rod inside the thigh bone with three screws at the hip and two at the knee. What a great way to start your senior year, with a walker! And hundreds of miles away from my hometown in New Jersey. This rod had held up pretty good over the years!

My anticipation grew as I waited for the doctor to come into the room. I was finally going to have an answer! With a big smile, I was kicking my feet like a little girl.

Oh, the PA came in, okay I guess. I had great interactions with PAs in grad school, I thought. He did a basic evaluation and asked the same questions I would have to an athlete. Well, that was uneventful, I thought. I felt a little deflated but I was still amped up about what the doctor would tell me.

If the PA was the plateau then this is where it went downhill. The doctor came in and looked at the x-rays and said they were fine, that I had arthritis and in so many words told me I needed to suck it up. I felt panicked. My head slowly started to spin. I explained to him that the pain was deep inside the middle of my joint. I was active and now I'm not. I told him my pain tolerance was high and this was painful, 10/10! I politely suggested an MRI. He argued back it would be no use because I had three screws in the hip and the image wouldn't be good. I said it could still show something worth viewing. He grudgingly gave me a script. I was exhausted and felt belittled and like I was a liar. I couldn't wait to get that MRI to prove him wrong. Then he'd have to help me.

One problem with that scenario: I never heard from him again. He never called to update me on the results, he never followed up. I called once with no return call.

I didn't know until years later, when I was creating a course for others with RA that this was called gaslighting. The impact was devastating to me for years to come.

Two years went by. I lost my confidence in knowing my body. I lost trust in medical professionals. These were my people! How could that be? My head was spinning with absolute confusion. Was I really now

a wimp? Did RA lower my pain tolerance so much that I couldn't handle a little pain or dysfunction? Did I even have anything that bad? Was I making this all up in my head? Was I any good at evaluating my own patients?

Two years I spent defeated and feeling like I was in an alternate reality. I was in bad shape and getting worse, barely walking, barely sleeping, barely doing anything. I changed my clothing and shoes to accommodate. I stopped going out with my friends as much. I kept my mouth shut about the pain I felt. I just ignored the impairments. But a year after the fateful visit, my rheumatologist saw me worsening and sent me to get a cortisone shot. This led me to a holistic doctor, an osteopathic doctor. I was also going to an acupuncturist and a physical therapist. All were just keeping me above the water enough to not drown. I was using two canes at work, depending on student workers to do any lifting and longer walking. I was getting three hours of sleep a night, if I was lucky. I feared vicodin addiction and life in a hospital bed. My life was horrible, I hated my body betraying me so badly. My weight was down to a scarce 102 pounds. And the only path looked like hospice. I was in disbelief that a 34 year old, otherwise healthy, loving-life individual could be so condemned. But I trusted the opinion of the higher medical professional.

Then one day as I crutched my way into the athletic training room, exhausted from the walk into work, I saw my team physician. He was shocked as he looked at me and asked how long I had been like this. I said two years. He couldn't believe he had missed seeing this. He told me I needed to get to his office ASAP. Oh my! I was so relieved! Finally someone believes me! Finally some action!

He told me that the x-rays taken two years ago were non-weight bearing and that should never have been done like that. "You can't see joint space accurately like that," he stated. My new x-rays looked rough and he told me I needed surgery. Although I was scared to death he made me cry with joy. This was further validated by my surgeon when he said my hip looked like brown sugar and water and that I was two years late! I was mad at myself. I was disappointed I didn't trust myself. I believed an authority, I trusted him and he betrayed my trust. I suffered mentally and physically because I didn't empower myself. Lesson learned, all too well. Now I am a Wyld Chyld. A boss of my body babe!

Pooja Panchamia

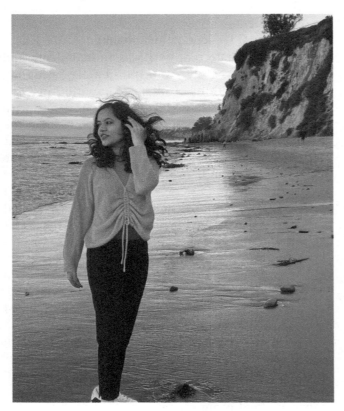

"The quote that keeps me going during tough times is the one by Dumbledore: 'Happiness can be found, even in the darkest of times, if only one remembers to turn on the light.' It is not the feeling of happiness (remission in this case) in itself, but the pursuit and the journey of finding that light and hope that pushes us out of the dark. Always remember to turn on that light."

One morning in August 2017, I woke up from the bed but could not move my legs. My knees were stiff and there was a bizarre numbness and tingling in my feet that I had never felt before. It became a new routine for the next few weeks - waking up with rigid joints, struggling to start the day, rushing to the office, and being fatigued by the end of the day. Balancing my health and work was not alien to me, I had been doing it since childhood while coping with asthma. But this was new. This was unpredictable. When I was finally making strides with living healthier, trekking 45 miles, and running 10Ks, I felt betrayed that my body could not keep up. Like taking one step forward, two steps backward.

While there were some dismissal experiences initially, where doctors misconstrued my joint pain as nutrition deficiency, I am thankful to our family physician who suspected rheumatoid arthritis (RA), which was later confirmed through blood work. However, in those 10-12 weeks, my stiffness and pain had spread to my fingers, which affected my daily chores and ability to type at work. Until then, I had not mentioned anything to my friends and colleagues, as I had absolutely no idea what was happening in my body and why it was functioning the way it was. I cannot imagine the trauma people suffer due to late diagnosis and treatment. My diagnosis was followed by fear of the unknown, anxiety, and denial. Due to a lack of awareness, I always associated the word 'arthritis' with old age. At 24, this diagnosis was heart-wrenching. Imagine, you are living your best life, loving the work that you do, feeling fit, exploring the world, and you come down with an autoimmune condition that is lifelong with no proven cause or cure. In India, there is also some stigma associated with 'being young and sick'. 'Invisible disability' is a term that most people have never heard of. As an introvert, I often bottled up emotions and would not easily seek help, so it took everything in my power to open up about my illness and emotions – to my doctors, family, friends, and colleagues. RA was also humbling in so many ways. A prideful person who hated coming off as weak, I had to ask for help for the most basic tasks such as opening a bottle.

It was not easy, I felt guilty all the time – guilty for missing a close friend's birthday, guilty for not being there for my family, guilty for missing office dinners, and guilty for being self-obsessed. I was exhausted from explaining to people why I don't feel good, and I resorted to making excuses that were easier to communicate. In a matter of weeks, I went through a roller-coaster of emotions - lonely, fearful, misunderstood, and disconnected. I felt grief for the life I had. I wasn't bogged down by the illness as much as the uncertainty of how it will change the course of my life. Of course, doctors asked me to stop googling my symptoms. But nobody would sit me down and explain the severity, risks, and new reality of my life. They asked me to accept and not fight the diagnosis, but what am I accepting here? One night while I was listening to the Fight song by Rachel Platten, I felt as if the song was written for me and decided to finally steer the direction of my life. *"Starting right now I'll be strong, I'll play my fight song, And I don't really care if nobody else believes, Cause I've still got a lot of fight left in me."* It was an aha moment for me.

Starting that day, I did three things. Since I was feeling extremely dependent, I decided to take my first solo trip. My parents were petrified of me traveling alone, but it was essential for my own mental peace. I went to Cambodia for five days. I grappled with stiffness after sitting for hours or walking a long distance, and struggled with carrying my luggage. But I felt a breath of fresh air. The ability to manage despite these limitations and fend for myself boosted my confidence and self-esteem. Watching the sunrise over Angkor Wat, and sitting in a Buddhist monastery, slowly erased all the memories of distress and discomfort. It was like meditation, soaking in the sun while imagining a new life. I wouldn't say I had accepted my condition, but it was the first step in that direction.

Second, I came to the realization that I am not the only person in the world who is dealing with such a new normal. I reached out to a few RA patient advocates and bloggers on Twitter and listened to their life stories. These wonderful people alleviated my uncertainty and helped me look beyond my disease, and that is when I decided to start 'FieryBones,' an online autoimmune arthritis patient community. FieryBones shares stories and provides a social community to people balancing their lives, chasing dreams, and managing parenthood while simultaneously battling their chronic diseases. Stories healed me, and I wanted to pass that comfort to other patients as they are learning to cope. As the community continues to touch the lives of thousands of people, it is messages like these that bring me joy and warms my heart:

> *"Stories on FieryBones hit me hard as it is somewhere my story too. Thank you for making me believe I am not alone, and this illness does not define me."*

As much as I Hate this illness, I am grateful to it for defining my purpose in healthcare.

Third, I decided to be kind to myself. Especially when your symptoms are not visible, other people may not always understand what you are going through. Hence, I feel a deeper need to express appreciation to myself for all the things that I manage independently – multiple doctor appointments, weekly self-injecting medication, therapy, business school, and life in a foreign country. Each day is different. On good days, I am an extra productive ball of energy, who wants to be everywhere and do everything, because, in the back of my head, I know the winter (bad days) is coming. It is a continuous cycle. No matter what people say about always staying happy, not taking stress, and living in the present – it is almost impossible to live that way. Instead, I am learning to understand my pattern of emotions. During every flare, I know I am going to feel low and anxious about not being able to live the life I want. Sometimes when the medications start working and you begin to feel good, you instinctively expect that feeling to linger. But in these last five years, I have experienced many ups and downs. While each down has devastated me, each up is what I look forward to. Everyone finds a coping mechanism, and for me, dark humor has been an escape. The chronic community is pretty entertaining on social media where I end up laughing over relatable memes. I refer to my immune system as the third person many times, while joking about how it is so dumb to mistake my joints as a foreign body, how it has gone into over-active mode again and needs to take a chill pill, or how it is the product of my faulty genes.

As an ardent Harry Potter fan, for me, living with RA is like tasting Bertie Bott's Every Flavor Beans. Some days are as sweet and delicious as Cherry and Green Apple, while others are as terrifying as Dirt or Booger, and you have absolutely no idea which one you are going to pick. It might seem that life is falling apart, but if all the pieces come back together, wouldn't life become too boring? You need to look forward to something, you need the bad days to fully appreciate the good ones. The quote that keeps me going during tough times is the one by Dumbledore – *"Happiness can be found, even in the darkest of times, if only one remembers to turn on the light."* It is not the feeling of happiness (remission in this case) in itself, but the pursuit and the journey of finding that light and hope that pushes us out of the dark. Always remember to turn on that light.

Mariam Aslam

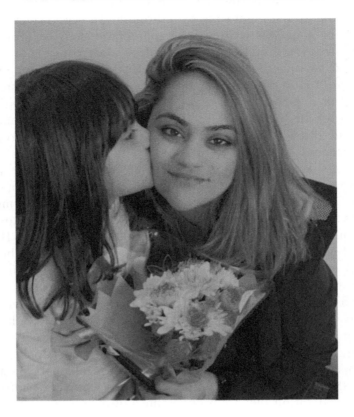

"Live your best life with rheumatoid arthritis!"

"You have rheumatoid arthritis, and there is no cure," the doctor said as she walked back into the cold room with my diagnosis. I was shocked and in disbelief, as I drove home without a care plan and an unwillingness to figure it out. No one talked about how it would feel. I started isolating myself, so I wouldn't have to answer anyone's questions about what was happening to me. It became difficult to think about anything other than the excruciating pain.

RA impacted my life in ways I couldn't imagine. I began having trouble with simple tasks like brushing my teeth and getting a good night's sleep. Being unable to take care of myself led me to a poor quality of life, and the pain only worsened from there. I lost mobility in two major joints and my self-esteem was at an all-time low. All I could think of was what people would think when they saw my swollen, crooked fingers. I realized that I would need to adjust my mindset to manage my RA and live a more wholesome, happy life. I had to figure out how to eliminate the sinking depression and lack of self-esteem.

With an ounce of willingness, I booked my first therapy session. At first, it was hard to open up about what I was really feeling. I am continuously learning coping strategies with my therapist to solve current problems. I constantly remind myself to get out of the negative thoughts. Keeping up with my mental health has helped me improve how I care for myself physically. I believe that true healing begins when you accept yourself for who you are, mentally and physically. I discovered that shifting my mindset helped me become a hopeful RA warrior and live my best life with RA.

Lisa Hobock

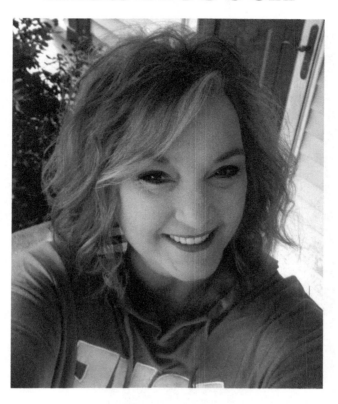

"Pain is a journey. You will go through tunnels, dead-ends and many paths. Stay strong so no matter what, you never lose your way."

My story goes from joy to deep depression. For years I knew something was wrong physically but it took years to find the right doctor who believed me and did testing. I was relieved, but also sad to find out. I grieved for the person I physically used to be. I was sad because I could no longer do things I used to do.

Before my symptoms and the pain became so bad I took for granted so much. I would see my friends going and doing things and instead I would be in bed in tears because my pain was out of control. So the depression got worse.

I'm thankful that I have a wonderful rheumatologist and she treats my physical pain as well as mental health. So I'm having more good days than bad ones. It's a journey that is never ending, but today I'm thankful for the little things.

Dominique Richmond

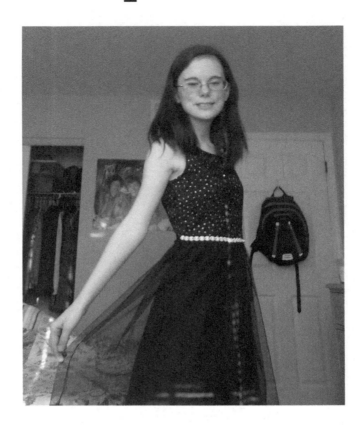

"Juvenile arthritis is no fun, but you will get through it. One step at a time."

I was diagnosed with JIA on May 10th, 2019 when I was 14 years of age. I know that doesn't sound young, but me being in middle school, already having the symptoms of it and doctors couldn't tell me what was happening, it was hard. It was a life changing diagnosis. Sure, I was already diagnosed with anxiety but that didn't change anything. When I saw my amazing rheumatologist, she had no idea if mine would be long or short term. But I'm lucky that I also met my amazing therapist outside of school.. She helped me understand more about the diagnosis. She helped me process what was going through my head.

Medicine was difficult. I was on so many it wasn't funny. My iron was low, I still have to take iron supplements. Vitamin D and C was low, still taking those supplements. My inflammation was high, so my doctor started me on methotrexate and Celebrex. I had to stop the methotrexate because it bothered my stomach and Celebrex caused me gastritis, though it might not for you. Then I had to change to enbrel. It worked but then I had pain after using it for so long. On top of that I was on leflunomide. And now I'm on a humira injection. That was a lot to cope with. It was so many medication changes, shots in my legs, finding some of them I can't tolerate. I was breaking down because of the methotrexate. I was on eight pills before the injection. I was gagging every time I tried to take my medication later on. Then we just quit after the injection. But it's overwhelming.

Middle school was horrible, I was pushed around, shoved into lockers and was called grandma. I had an IEP (individualized education plan) so me and my "team", who was in charge of my IEP, put an accommodation saying I could leave five minutes early. It was a big middle school. The bullying didn't stop. I was asked many times why I was allowed to leave early and why I didn't wait for the bell. I couldn't respond, I didn't know how, nor did I want to tell them why. I cried about it a lot to my school counselor on how unfair it was and how my art teacher didn't understand me. It was awful.

Then High School came. There are two high schools on the road where I go to school. We have a regular senior high school then we have an alternative high school. I'm at the alternative because of my disabilities. I have a lot. And I met a new school counselor, who was just as amazing. She listened, let me cry and did weekly check-ins to make sure I was okay. Mentally I wasn't.

Covid sucked. While people were getting their Covid shots because they are high risk, I was at home with Covid. My symptoms came on very slowly. Then I was quarantined for months because my whole family got it, making it more of a high risk.

My coping mechanism for this was to keep it hidden from some people. I told my friends because I knew them for a while, but I kept it a little bit of a secret from my counselors as long as I could till I had enough. I told my ex girlfriend right away because I needed to get it off my chest. And she kept it a secret. I unfortunately had no choice not to keep it a secret when it came to teachers. And in ninth grade, I was still coping, trying to accept myself.

The only way I was able to finally accept myself was to do my favorite hobbies, which is, singing, dancing, writing songs and books, playing piano and so much more. And talking to my out of school therapist every month, I was slowly getting there. It wasn't that long ago, maybe a year or so, I finally accepted myself. I finally did. Somedays I wouldn't wish this upon my worst enemy because of my immune system. But I got through it.

If I had something to say to someone who is new to having arthritis and is young, like younger than 18, you're not alone. You're not. It might feel like it but it's okay. You can follow the Arthritis Foundation on Instagram and meet a lot of people with juvenile arthritis. You've got this. I believe in you! Stay strong out there! Juvenile arthritis is no fun, but you will get through it. One step at a time.

Cristina Montoya

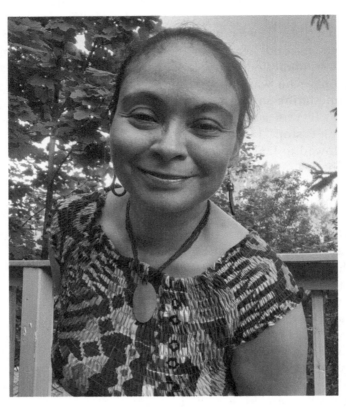

"I truly believe in the saying that when you smile, the whole world smiles with you. Sure, there are hardships, sad moments, times when you feel like giving up. But look at all the meaningful connections you've made in spite of RA – and even because of it. I wouldn't have some of the most amazing friends if it wasn't for my rheumatic condition. They give me a sense of solidarity. I find comfort in chatting with them, talking about my symptoms and having the whole room nod in approval, "Yes, me too."

I grew up in Medellin, Colombia, where I followed a healthy lifestyle such as exercising regularly and eating wholesome, fresh food. Despite my lifestyle, at 22 years of age, I was diagnosed with rheumatoid arthritis (RA) and Sjogren's syndrome. I had a quick onset of the disease, so my RA was diagnosed within two months.

The disease was so aggressive, my fingers became deformed within six months of diagnosis.

The era of biologics was in its early stages and completely inaccessible to me due to financial reasons. Lifting a sheet of paper, or typing in my last research paper, hurt like hell. I was terrified of not being able to graduate as a nutritionist and dietitian with my peers. Thanks to a load of corticosteroids, I reached the finish line.

Fast forward, one of my most traumatic experiences since my RA diagnosis happened was when my rheumatologist strongly advised me against becoming a mom in my late 20's. For years, I thought I was infertile.

When I suddenly became pregnant at 36, my heart sank because I was still on methotrexate. Several doctors suggested termination, but I believed my baby had a purpose in this world. I reached out to an RA patient advocate who referred me to a facebook support group called "Mamas Facing Forward." I've found a rheumatologist specializing in infertility in Toronto. The specialist's office was right across the street from my rheumatologist's office. Irony?

The specialist explained that while it was not advisable to conceive on methotrexate, because of the increased chance of miscarriage and congenital deformities by 7%, I still had a 93% chance of having a healthy child. Focus on the 93%, he said. I received excellent care from this rheumatologist and fetal medicine specialist during my pregnancy. I was not expecting to face yet another health challenge.

My rheumatologist said I would have an arthritis flare 8-10 weeks postpartum. But just one day after delivering, I had a full-force RA attack, which showed my body no mercy. I felt as though 1,000 flaming needles poked my entire body. It was the kind of pain that made me doubt my abilities as a new mother. I refused narcotics; I wanted to be alert for my baby. The nurses did everything they could to help me feed him. We all failed miserably.

The pain from breastfeeding was so unbearable that the incision from my c-section felt like a paper cut. On top of that, I wasn't producing enough milk, and my baby's blood sugar was dropping. I had no choice but to supplement with the "F" word (i.e., formula). And despite their attentiveness to my son and me, the maternity ward staff dismissed the excruciating pain I suffered from my RA.

My flare-up caused congestive heart failure and pulmonary edema (i.e. fluid in the lungs), forcing me to leave my two-week-old newborn at home while I stayed in the hospital.

Hopelessness and despair invaded my whole being. While I learned that motherhood was more than just breastfeeding, all the little things I had to do for my son – changing his diaper, bathing him, pushing his stroller – took out of me the little energy I had left. I went from being a "high-risk"

pregnancy case to a nobody in the healthcare system. I had poor access to mental and physical support on how to care for my child while living with chronic pain.

Fortunately, my husband flew my mom in from Colombia to Canada a month before my boy was born. We have an old tradition where moms look after their daughters for 40 days after giving birth. A period called "La dieta or cuarentena," which means quarantine. It is a time when new moms must invest 100% of their time in recovering, resting, and learning about their new role as a mom.

I was lucky to have a wonderful social and family network to support me during my first six months postpartum. Otherwise, I would likely not be in this world. The five stars treatment I received during my pregnancy dropped to zero after giving birth.

After surviving the postpartum pain and, most recently, a Covid-19 infection, I am reminded that living with rheumatoid arthritis is a marathon, not a sprint. We must focus on what we CAN control. Self-advocacy is our most powerful tool if we want to thrive with RA.

Self-advocacy became a vital tool to overcome barriers to accessing quality care. I couldn't just wait for the services to come to my house. When I was re-hospitalized, a kind pregnant female rheumatologist assessed me at the ER. Her bed-side-manner was excellent and I begged her to take me as a patient. I wish there were more women in rheumatology. After three painful years, three different biologics and a Covid-19 infection, my RA seems to be under better control.

Don't let rheumatoid arthritis overshadow your inner beauty and life projects. Sure, you will need to make changes and adapt. This disease also teaches us to be more resilient and stronger individuals. The old saying, it takes a village to raise a child, also applies to people living with RA. Build your village, surround yourself with supportive friends and family who will be there for you, no matter the pain and unexpected complications.

Karen Gray

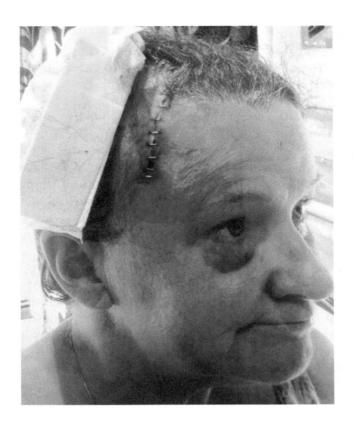

"When they say 'it's all in your head' never, ever believe it."

My story begins, not with rheumatoid arthritis, but with a tumor in my head and a doctor who, for over eight years, believed there was nothing physically wrong with me and that my headaches, etc were 'all in my head'. She was wrong. Eventually it was discovered I had a tumor and it was removed - all good.

As I lay in that hospital bed I was overcome with an indescribable rapturous joy that I was, finally, at last, to be pain free for the first time in over ten years.

However, the trauma my body went through and, I believe, the inflammation that was consistent within my head for weeks after, caused my body to go 'askew' and I developed rheumatoid arthritis - something I had never even heard of.

I now live with pain every day. My expected 'joy' has been destroyed - I am crushed. I will never be free of it. My challenge: To free my mind of its pain.

SOCIAL LIFE & RELATIONSHIPS

Stories

Judith Flanagan

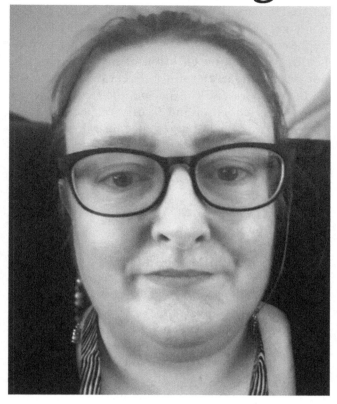

"Connect with others, be kind to yourselves and each other, do what works for you treatment wise, say no when you need to, find your tribe for support whether online or offline. Support is key; nobody has to do this alone."

Diagnosis

I was diagnosed with seropositive rheumatoid arthritis in 2012. My general practitioner at the time suspected it and sent me for some blood tests. The blood tests showed a high rheumatoid factor so he then sent me to a rheumatologist to get some x-rays, which were carried out by the radiologist. My x-rays and blood tests were viewed by the rheumatologist and the diagnosis of seropositive rheumatoid arthritis was given.

What initially lead to the Diagnosis.

In 2010 I had unexplained injuries. An unexplained type of pain caused me to fall to the ground. I couldn't walk, I was on crutches after going to the hospital with my family. I had no idea how it happened or why it happened. In 2012 I was studying at an educational institution called TAFE, where more symptoms began their attack.

Symptoms that led me to my local General Practitioner and then Rheumatologist.

My hands started to swell to the point I couldn't lift or move computers or play around with computer parts. I also began limping around TAFE and I had to walk from home to TAFE and back home from bus stops. I couldn't put my trousers on and off and struggled putting my shoes and socks on.

I rarely went to the doctor. My family convinced me to go and I was rather concerned so off I went to my local medical center. My foster mum came along with me. Ever since living with this disease visits to the GP, and specialist care teams, are a regular part of life and something we have to keep on top of.

Advocating for Oneself.

After I was diagnosed I began my own facebook page called United Advocacy Australia. I wanted to share resources from other organizations as well as creating my own graphics in support of all who live with arthritis. I'd later learned that there are over 100 forms of arthritis. I began looking for some organizations and nonprofits that focused on either multiple chronic illnesses or arthritis conditions. I found two that sparked my interest and I wanted to get involved by volunteering, which then helped me in learning about not just my conditions but also support and resources for other forms.

How I Advocate By Using My Voice And Sharing My Insights.

- I am an arthritis representative;
- A patient partner with the International Pain Foundation;
- These are the main two I have had a lot of involvement with and have regularly participated in awareness campaigns and projects with, since 2013 and onwards.

- I have been a contributor in a few of the IPain Living Magazines;
- I am a co-host in some episodes in the Arthritis Voices 360 podcast;
- I have participated in research by completing surveys;
- I have been an admin for the AiArthritisVoices website;
- I have been an admin for a community team research project;
- I have been involved in the book "Real Life Diaries, Living With Rheumatic Disease";
- I'm a #CureArthritisCrew member with the Arthritis National Research Foundation;
- I am a #BreakthroughCrew member with Clara Health for my support of clinical trials;
- A Wego Health patient leader;
- A Savvy Coop Co-Owner

Finding Your Tribe.

Finding your tribe for support is super important. Someone who understands your ups and also your downs, someone who lives with your condition and understands your treatments, why you take them and how it affects your overall health. A support group either online, or in person, is an absolute must. You will in time get to learn what works for one doesn't work for all, but you can get a general idea of what is out there and can consult with your personalized health care teams. Always remember, we are the ones who live everyday with our conditions, and any complications that come with them, and anyone who cares for us needs to work with us in any decisions made regarding our care.

Invisible Illness and Invisible Disability.

Rheumatoid arthritis can have both physical and invisible ailments to it, like fatigue and even pain, that are very often misunderstood. Which is why I like to design my own graphics, outlining the invisible symptoms which are much more than pain, and support many projects and awareness activities wherever I can. Rheumatoid arthritis is a form of disability because it is a very debilitating condition that has many invisible symptoms and is why I will continue raising awareness through the projects I am involved in.

Pregnancy and Children.

On this very subject I have always felt so much pressure to have children but I decided very early on that I personally wasn't going there. I mean don't get me wrong, I love children, my nieces, nephew etc, but with everything that goes on health wise having children of my own just was not on my radar and not a direction I wanted to go in. I understand if other people take that road, that's their decision and I fully respect that, but I have always felt judged because I don't own my own home, or have a family of my own. It's just how society has always been. I don't have any regrets at all. I take my hat off to parents out there, I truly do, and even more so if you are someone who lives with a chronic condition. Amazing humans that is all.

Setting Boundaries.

You may feel obligated at times to do certain duties in life, but people who love you and support you will truly understand when you need to set your boundaries. The same goes for advocacy too if you need to take a break from projects, or take a break from being online you can. You can say no. I am here to tell you that it's perfectly ok and your tribe, whether online or in person, will still be there when you come back.

Knowing Your Worth. You may feel that what you have to say doesn't matter, or that you don't have much to say at all, but however you use your voice or share your insights it all matters. I used to think the same thing, however if I can help just one person through everything I do, then it can mean so much and maybe not just one person but many.

Connecting with Others.

My suggestion is that if someone is newly diagnosed, follow organizations related to arthritis and chronic illness, join support groups online or offline, watch webinars, read books and magazines, join forums, join chats, find orgs where you can volunteer from home to learn more and be in the know. If you are into clinical trials, maybe join one of those, attend conferences, either in person or online, to learn from professionals and people living with the condition, and listen to podcasts or medical talk shows.

Unsolicited Medical Advice.

Quite often suggestions will be made and they mean well, but in the end you will do what's right for you. You will.

Make an informed decision based on your healthcare team and current treatments available. Rheumatoid arthritis is treated with NSAIDS(non steroidal anti inflammatory drugs), DMARDS and biologics. Others may take different paths. DMARDS stands for disease modifying anti-rheumatic drugs, which are the first line of defense when treating rheumatoid arthritis. What works for one person doesn't mean it works the same for everyone; it can truly be trial and error.

My First Treatments.

My first treatments in 2012 were sulphasalazine, corticosteroid, methotrexate and plaquenil. I later went off plaquenil and steroids and went on humira. Humira didn't help at all and I was on that for a year, then from 2014 to 2020 I went on to actemra infusion via IV administered by a nurse. In 2020 I went on to the actemra pen which I could conveniently self administer from home.

The Covid Pandemic.

The Covid pandemic hit and I had to keep connecting with my pharmacist via an app, to check if I could get my treatment via the pen, as there was a worldwide shortage of actemra. I honestly struggled with the needle versions and it's why I preferred the pen. Throughout this pandemic I have lived on edge and felt rather stressed, not knowing whether I would be able to get my treatment or not. It's been a few close calls and I personally have skipped a couple to try and make it last between appointments. I always asked my rheumatologist at the time with a phone call. I may change at my next appointment cause it's all been so stressful.

My takeaway message to everyone who reads, please support and connect with others, be kind to yourselves and each other. Do what works for you treatment wise, say no when you need to, find your tribe for support, whether online or offline. Support is key; nobody has to do this alone.

McKayla Triffo

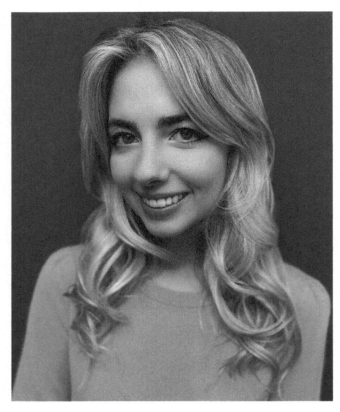

"We are valuable and needed: onscreen, onstage, at every table."

I Want to Play

"*What do you want to be when you grow up?*" A question we all know and have answered hundreds of times throughout our lives. In kindergarten, I wanted to be a princess. Of all my chosen professions, this one was somehow the most realistic of the gamut. I later desperately wanted to be an astronaut. It was my dearest dream to colonize the moon, and I even wrote brilliant elementary level literature on how to make it happen. I held fast to this vision up until I was diagnosed with the big juvenile rheumatoid arthritis bang. I was then informed that riding a rocket catapulting through the roaring G-Force, and leaving our home atmosphere, would kill or seriously harm me. My dream was crushed, and thus my old fervor for space has since been buried. After that, I wanted to be a drummer, or a dancer, because I love music and the fine arts. As my joint damage speedily progressed and I began to lose mobility in my hands, wrists, and eventually my legs, I gave up on those dreams too.

Among all my squashed dreams, there is one remaining eternally tattooed on my soul, no matter how many times doctors tell me that it is unattainable for me. I want to be included. It sounds like a shockingly boring, mundane, and easily accomplished (for most) goal. But it is in fact more difficult to achieve than one might anticipate, and this has been the bane of my existence, the desire that has brought about all of my dreadfully ridiculous circumstances that have since commenced: the aching yearn for normalcy.

I distinctly recall the incident that incited this goal in my heart. It was shortly after my diagnosis in third grade, and I found myself on the sidelines at recess. A favorite game among my peers was Red Rover, in which players lock hands, are charged at full-force, and tackled by a tough person trying to break the chain. My gnarly purple fingers were way too swollen and painful to hold hands, let alone sustain that kind of jarring. I asked to play another game and was met with confused laughter. I sat on the sidelines alone, and nobody thought to stick up for me. All of my able-bodied peers supported one another in the notion that it is more normal and okay for me to sit out alone, than make a change that slightly impacts everyone, because after all, I was only one person, and everyone else mattered more. After that, they did not even invite me to play games that I was physically able to. You need to stay on the sidelines. That is your role. Watching ballet practice, or my friends at recess, from the sidelines in a wheelchair is humbling in the worst way – especially when there are so many Olympians out there 'overcoming' their arthritis diagnosis and accomplishing athletic feats I could only come close to in my dreams. I was too sick. A failure. I could never be anyone's poster child success story, because arthritis overcame me, not the other way around.

In college, I studied theater. I have learned the inflexible plastic nature of the world of acting, yet it has remained stuck to the wall of my heart like gum on a stop sign. I was in a group working on a project in a lighting and sound course. We were kindred spirits, discussing plans to start filming comedy sketches and embark on a creative journey together. Many of them were known for advocating for social justice efforts on campus, so I got too comfortable and opened up about my fear of the critical eye of the camera capturing a profound deformity on one of my fingers. I would lose my security blanket by skillfully masking my visible baggage. One girl burst out laughing when I showed her. She said, *"oh my god, that looks like a fat grape that's about to pop!"* I remember standing there, aghast even after years of being sick and shouldering insensitive comments. I showed a group that was supposed to be understanding, evidence of my intimate struggle with a horrifically painful disease. They just laughed, and the group disbanded. We never made a comedy sketch. No members of the group spoke to me after that. I later received a partially cosmetic operation on that finger, due to that comment.

After the ugly finger debacle and numerous similar disheartening incidents, I unofficially retired from acting. I could no longer bear alone the unspeakable emotional burden of being the only person demanding inclusion and equitable treatment for myself and others like me. Being forced to the sidelines, after sticking up for myself, or trying to pull up a chair at a table I was not invited to, has been a common theme, a lesson society has tried to teach me numerous times. I could tell a million sob stories about how beaten down I have been, how many times I have almost let that narrative win. I have often allowed myself to believe that everyone on earth is ableist and there is no amount of education that can fix how deeply selfish people are. But, while the hurtful moments are important and contain lessons about why advocacy is so fundamental for disability rights, they are not the most meaningful. The most impactful stories show the bits of light, the moments that teach that not everyone is this way, even if it feels like it sometimes.

In 2019, I was at rock bottom after recovering from two grueling and deeply traumatizing back-to-back surgeries. I was barely making it through the day as a substitute teacher and I felt acutely alone and unfulfilled. One day, scrolling on social media, I saw an open call audition for a play that is dear to my heart. After allowing the angel and devil on my shoulders to heatedly debate, I caved and sent in a half–hearted video audition at the last minute. I did not expect a response, but sure enough, I got a call back. After that, I was cast — and terrified. Professional stage acting is no joke,

and the grueling physical undertaking made me worry I would not be able to see my role through. I panicked that I had made a horrible decision. One evening, I had no choice but to go to the hospital for an alarming symptom. My biggest fear was possible repercussions of missing rehearsal the next day. The lack of anger from the cast and crew was unlike anything I had experienced before. I was flabbergasted at the heartfelt reaction and care. After that, the ladies who were performing alongside me formed a circle of protection and encouragement around me. I remember once, in a rare moment of sharing trust, I expressed concern about costuming to a cast-mate and I was so frightened to ask for what I needed, because of being punished for doing that in the past. She imparted great wisdom to me: *"we all have needs. You should not be afraid to ask for what you need just because you think it is somehow different and an undue burden. You are an important part of this show. You need to be on stage to tell this story. People who see your value will know that and give you what you need. It is a small price for them to pay."*

I had not realized how long I had spent being undervalued. Most importantly, I had not realized that there are people out there who care for others and have the capacity to value me.

During the Covid pandemic I have experienced a turbulent sea of emotions, and I would be lying if I said I did not revert to my prior feelings about society after watching how selfish and dismissive even some of my most beloved relations were to people like me. Like in Red Rover, others wanted me to sacrifice my physical and mental wellness for theirs. They were repulsed by the notion of making a small change in their personal lives to protect mine, how horrible and harmful to do anything to show that disabled lives are worth living and worth protecting.

But even so, my high risk peers and others online rose up in droves to face that violence. Even during the hardest days, I was simultaneously re-learning that I am not alone after all. There are so many more chronically ill and disabled folks out there than I realized, and I only could not see them because of the same barriers to access that I have been battling my whole life. There are others out there who will fight for disability rights, even if they are not always in the same room as me. Expanding this movement starts with advocacy and education.

Because we are valuable and needed: onscreen, onstage, at every table.

Ashley Krivohlavek

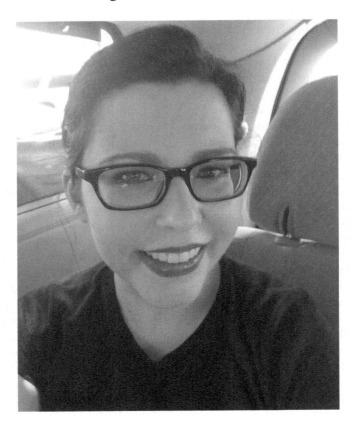

"Feeling like life is going on without you is one of the most difficult feelings we as humans face. As an immunosuppressed person during a pandemic, it has been very difficult to be social and keep up in a world that seems to be moving on, even if I can't."

In late February 2020, my friend had her annual birthday party for all of her friends. We went to a restaurant and the pub across the street. I distinctly remember everyone taking guesses when we would be able to get back together again. I thought by summer we would be back to our regular get-togethers.

Eight years ago, I was diagnosed with psoriatic arthritis (PsA). I have had psoriasis (PsO) since I was twelve and it was under control. The PsA was a complete surprise. One night I went to bed and the next, I couldn't walk. Literally overnight, my entire life had changed. I have been familiar with autoimmune diseases since I can remember. My maternal grandfather had rheumatoid arthritis (RA) and my maternal aunt had lupus. My mother has had osteoarthritis (OA) for at least thirty years and has been diagnosed with RA since my own diagnosis.

When I first got diagnosed, I withdrew from everything and everyone. I didn't want to deal with what my life now entailed. Countless doctor's appointments, labs, endless time on the phone with insurance, the doctor's office and pharmacies. I didn't know anyone my age doing the things I was now required to do just to be able to move. For months, I withdrew and didn't speak about what I was going through.

After about six months, I knew I had to come to the surface, tell my story and offer what I had learned through my experience. I started talking and going out with my friends that I knew before my diagnosis. I started looking for platforms that offered socializing with other PsA patients. I signed up for Twitter and began to talk to patient organizations about volunteering my time. After I started opening up about my diagnosis and what was happening, so many offered their support and love.

After my diagnosis and prior to 2020, I would see my friends at least once a month. We went out to eat, watch movies, travel together and shop. However, my diagnosis meant that there were instances when I couldn't be there for my friends. A destination wedding that I couldn't attend because of a hospitalization, due to my lowered immune system, a family trip to Alaska that I couldn't go on because of a flare, many dinners that had to be postponed and being cautious about large get-togethers during flu and cold season. 2020 changed all of that.

In the last two years, I haven't seen many of my friends in person. I lost friends during the pandemic because of my inability to do many of the things we used to. 2020 felt like the time after I was newly diagnosed all over again. It was devastating for a social person like me to start all over again. Slowly, I began to strengthen my bonds with those that understood my disease. I spoke to my autoimmune friends through Twitter and we offered support and strength to each other. It helped to know that so many people were going through the same struggles. My in-person friends were supportive and would check in with me by text or zoom. We did zoom happy hours, we had group texts and tried to buoy each other.

Now, as Covid vaccinations are widely available and everything starts opening up, fear of the world moving on without me is becoming real again. I see my in-person friends going back to work, going out to eat in restaurants, get Covid and survive, date, go shopping and in general carry on with their lives in ways that I cannot. Feeling like life is going on without you is one of the most difficult feelings we as humans face. As an immunosuppressed person during a pandemic,

it has been very difficult to be social and keep up in a world that seems to be moving on, even if I can't.

If I could go back to my February 2020 life, I would give my pre-pandemic self some advice on friendships:

- Strengthen bonds with in-person friends and reinforce appreciation for their friendship.
- Strengthen bonds with the online community. They understand so much of what each other is going through.
- Don't withdraw. Reach out. I needed social interaction but, I erroneously assumed that everyone else was doing better than me and I needed to work on my needs myself. I quickly found out that so many felt the same as me.
- Be there for others. It puts your own issues in perspective when you are there for others.
- Recognize that you are different and it doesn't make your needs more or less important than others.
- Being a friend and having friends, while having PsA, requires a lot of patience and understanding from everyone. Just as I thought I had my disease and friendships balanced, a pandemic upended so much of what I built. However, through it all, I have met many people that are sharing my struggle, who love and support me. I love and support them too. When it is safe enough for all, we will all get together.

As I type this, my friend is again having her birthday. Two years later and I won't be there with her. I texted her for her birthday and sent her a gift to be delivered to her house. Even though I am not with her in person, I am thinking of her. For now, that's the best I can do and she knows and acknowledges that. I am proud to call her, and so many others, friends.

Joanne Schmoll

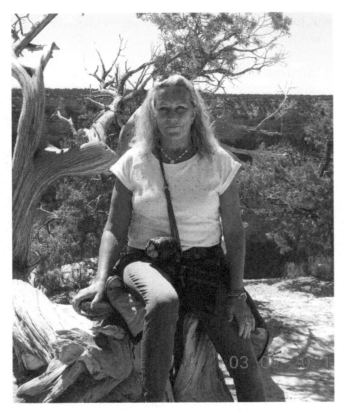

"Hearing others tell their story, and what they are doing to fight RA, is an inspiration."

I was diagnosed with RA in Sept 2020. I was 56 years old at that time. I had been having aches and pains with swelling in my hand and shoulder, hip, and knee pain. Sleep was becoming a problem although I was never a good sleeper. I was having arm and shoulder pain at night with tingling and numbness. It was hard to get comfortable. I was super tired all of the time. I woke up everyday with stiffness in my body.

I finally saw a rheumatologist, who did a complete work up with all the testing that goes with it. She put me on a high dose of prednisone for three to four weeks and all of my pain subsided temporarily. She diagnosed me with seronegative RA and said that I should start on hydroxychloroquine.

I didn't want to believe her. I didn't want to take those kinds of medications. I spoke to family members about my new diagnosis and no one seemed concerned. I looked ok but I felt terrible. Everyone seemed to think I had osteoarthritis and it was a normal process in aging. I tried to explain the difference but I think people thought I was just exaggerating or looking for attention. I thought maybe the doctor was wrong. Why would I have an autoimmune disease?

I refused the medication at first and tried changing my diet and adding supplements to my daily routine. The pain continued and I still wasn't getting any support from my family members. I was tired of hearing, *"everyone has aches and pains."* I was told by one person that I wouldn't know what pain was like until I was her age. She is thirteen years older than me and in good health. It was very stressful not having support with what I was going through. The tiredness was overwhelming.

Finally after almost a year, I decided I was going to have to fight this and believe it is real. It wasn't going to go away. I gave in and started the hydroxychloroquine. With the help from support groups online for RA, I'm finally beginning to accept my condition. It's nice to hear from people who can empathize with me. I get support to keep fighting and learn ways to help me feel better. Hearing others tell their story and what they are doing to fight RA is an inspiration. I read every RA article I can get my hands on. I take many supplements and try to stay on a healthy diet. I do not speak with family members about my condition anymore.

I have had some improvement with the swelling in my hand but I have stiffness now in both hands in the morning. My feet and ankles are starting to bother me now. I learned the more I move the better off I am. I learned that a good night's sleep is imperative. I'm so impressed with the RA warriors that I read about in the support groups and I will continue to fight this battle with their help.

If I can get off of this medicine someday I will be happy and if not, I won't feel discouraged. I will continue to fight and learn how to live with this.

Biz Brooks

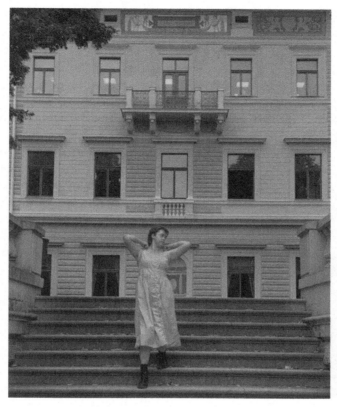

"No one around me understands the isolation and loneliness a teen goes through being disabled, having arthritis, and managing those two through a pandemic."

In sixth grade they told me my jaw joints disintegrated. In tenth grade I was diagnosed with arthritis, after multiple surgeries during the Covid pandemic. Despite being severely immunocompromised and isolated, I never noticed how lonely it made me feel. I didn't feel that aching in my chest to be a part of society, or that desperate plea to be allowed in, until it came to the 28th of February. 2022. I had attended in-person school before that date, with my non-disabled peers in the eleventh grade, while all of us wore masks and kept our distance. That Monday changed my experience. The mask mandate in my school building was lifted and it felt like a slap in the face. What about me? If I get sick, I go off of three of my meds and I'm out for weeks or maybe months. Do they care about disabled people? About people with arthritis? About me? I felt alone because of my illness for the first time. Can I still be a part of my community? Will my friends care enough to keep them on for me? Am I an inconvenience or infringing on others rights by asking that they protect my health and allow me to get the same education they can get?

All these questions ran through my head and still circulate my mind now. I still go to my high school but am always hit with a twitch of fear and loneliness. No one around me understands the isolation and loneliness a teen goes through being disabled, having arthritis, and managing those two through a pandemic. I make art about this feeling. One in particular features a person naked but still wearing a mask, sitting among the brush. Their eyes are desperate and they shy away from the frame. Sometimes I see that person as me, in the crowded hallways of a mask-free high school.

Lawrence Phillips

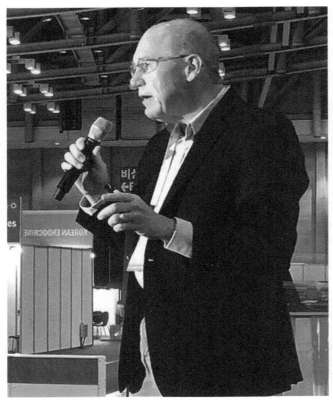

"It's lonely sometimes."

I was diagnosed with type 1 diabetes at age 17. While that age is a little older than average, it is still part of the age group where it is most likely to be diagnosed. It is often misunderstood that type 1 diabetes is a childhood disease. It can be diagnosed at any age, and variants of the disease have shown up in people as late as their 70s. But the statistical average is that people aged 25, or less, are most likely to be diagnosed, with birth to age 14 the age to be diagnosed.

While I was not diagnosed until I was 17, type 1 diabetes was part of my entire life. My mother was diagnosed when she was 23, and in those days, diabetes was a much more difficult disease than when I was diagnosed some 12 or so years later. Those 12 years between the time of each diagnosis were traumatic for my family. My mother's many complications meant that the family was always on edge. We often felt she would die any second and it stressed us, (my father and I), to the extreme.

During those 12 years, it was assumed that I would be diagnosed with diabetes at some point. Medical science misunderstood the familial connection of diabetes from parent to child. What was known was that children of a person with type 1 diabetes were at greater risk of having the disease than the regular population. For that reason, I had to take a glucose tolerance test every year. That was a four hour test where I was required to drink a heavy sugary mix, and my blood glucose was tested with blood draws each hour. That test is awful even today but, unlike today, in the 1970s, it was the only early warning test parents had, to know if their child was in the initial phase of losing their ability to control blood sugar. While I passed (unlike in the 1960s, today we know blood sugar is not a pass-fail test) each year, the test communicated the certainty that I would have diabetes, not if.

All that pretesting, plus my mother's declining condition, meant that I assumed that someday my autoimmune system would turn on, attack, and destroy my body's ability to produce insulin. Therefore, when it happened, I was prepared for it*. I had been waiting, and at age 17, I thought I might get lucky and defy the odds. But the good part was I was already resigned to it when it came. Of course, I would not say I liked it, I hated taking insulin and I was angry about the opportunities that diabetes took from me. But unlike others my age and younger, I was resigned to the outcome before it ever happened.

As a result of that thinking and my exposure to people who had diabetes, that my mother met during her journey, I already had a social network of people with type 1 diabetes. I knew many, some my age and even younger, who had diabetes. I already understood much of the local community. So, when I joined the online community of people with diabetes around 2006, I felt right at home. It was an easy transition.

Things were much different for rheumatoid disease (RD). First, I did not expect that I might someday be diagnosed with RD. When I was diagnosed with RD in 2000, I was stunned. I asked the doctor to tell me his findings twice because I was not sure I had completely understood him. He looked at me with a face that told me he was annoyed that he had to take time to cover the material twice.

I was so dumbfounded I didn't even ask many questions. I absorbed the information and tried not to reflect my growing sense of disbelief as he talked about joint destruction. I wondered what he was talking about? I have diabetes; what did he mean I have something else? I was shocked.

After the appointment, I wanted to consult online sources to tell me this was not possible, or that surely the doctor had made the worst mistake. While having both diseases was not common, it turned out that it was certainly not unheard of. 25% of all people with one autoimmune disease develop a second.

I took the issue seriously and started treatment as soon as possible. Thankfully, due to my doctors being aggressive, I mostly managed RD well for about 15 years without the help of others. But when I decided to seek support from the online RD communities, I got my second shock.

Unlike the online diabetes community, I started participating in around 2006. The online RD community was three things.

1. Very supportive,
2. Only semi-active and most important,
3. All females; 95% or more of the online RD community is female.

Not surprisingly, it was challenging to find a male in the community. Therefore, any male who came into the community almost immediately was an outsider, and those who tried did not usually last long.

It is a fine line that males in the RD community walk. We must stay engaged even when issues do not pertain to us, and it behooves us to be our authentic selves but sometimes with great restraint. A good example is when a member complains about an issue with parental interference. If this were a male-dominated community, a person might say grow up and get over it. Yet such a coarse approach would never be tolerated in the RD community, which is a good thing.

This is quite different in the diabetes online community, where the ratio is about 60% female and 40% male. So, while I did find community, I also felt further isolation. It would have been easy to give up and go away. That is one of the reasons why most other men do not stay around.

Frankly, joining and being accepted by the community of people with RD was worth the effort to gain access. I realized I had two choices: I could stay in my isolation or find ways to reach out to the online community. So, after much thought, I decided to gamble, and I found myself reaching out. But how

to do it and still be genuine to me? The answer lay in thinking of myself as a servant leader.

I determined that the person who wants to be part of a community must first serve it. Servant leadership is a model that I admire. Robert Greenleaf advanced it and if you have interest, you can read about it in detail in the book, "Finding Leo" by Philip Mathew, and several other books written by Larry Spears.

So how could I serve? For instance, I could write guest posts for others who wanted content. I could also do podcast interviews and work to offer genuine support. It is a touchy balancing act. The key is that I had to be true to myself and valuable to the RD community.

Taking those steps is worth it to have friends who accept me and do not question my motives. I am a male in a female-dominated community. Do I want to control the community? Certainly not. Do I want to be the person who directs things? How could I? No, if I wish the fellowship of this community, I must serve it. I serve on the arthritis foundation local board of directors, write blog reviews, and write blogs where I can share my emotions and thoughts about RD.

In a male-dominated community, the one with the oversized ego is usually the leader. I have never been the toughest or the biggest, so leading has been difficult, even though I did it for many years in my job. In the RD and in the diabetes community, I find the one who exposes themselves as accurate is the one who is valued. To that end, I have found a home in the RD community. Not because I am always right or always in the mainstream; instead, I have found a way to serve, and that service has helped me to be accepted. So, my lesson about life in this community is to be real and to serve. Incidentally, those are great qualities for most of life in a chronic disease community, or life outside our communities. That attitude has helped me find many friends and I no longer feel alone. I hope you also can find the peace that comes from community.

*The reader should know that most of our thinking about familial passing of diabetes that we had in the 1960's was wrong. We know that each child of a person with type 1 diabetes has about a 25% chance of being diagnosed themselves. This is far from the 'when will it happen' thinking of my childhood. Thankfully, we know so much more today than we did 47 years ago when I was diagnosed.

Jed Finley

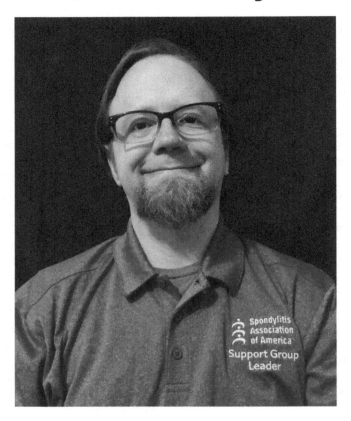

"People stop noticing you when you are in pain every day. Find a way to stay visible to the people around you."

The Red Cloak of Invisibility

Some time ago, I purchased three color coded wristbands from the National Ankylosing Spondylitis Society (NASS). They are: green for a good day, orange for an OK day, and red for a bad day.

The idea for them is that nobody will need to ask me how I'm doing because they simply need to look at my wrist.

As many people with chronic illness will tell you, one of the hardest parts of living the "Spoonie" life is always having to tell people how you're feeling. We get tired of needing to tell people multiple times a day, it forces us to think about our condition when we might not want to, and/or we need to deal with people who ask with a tone of, *"are you cured yet?"* It's a total pain in the butt (or back/legs/arms/feet/etc).

Because of the wrist bands I can avoid annoying or hurtful conversations. People can see I'm feeling crappy and they can give me space or accommodate for me.

In the beginning, it worked great! I wouldn't need to say anything but my team at school would know not to ask me to transport kids across campus, participate in PE, work on the ground, or any other more physically demanding tasks. I might get comments like *Oh, Jed's red today! Watch out.* But honestly, that didn't really bother me. I'd rather people be aware of my condition than think everything is fine and dandy!

For a while, my wrist displayed the full mix of different colors throughout the week. Rarely did I ever get a chance to wear green, but it still made a few appearances. Orange was standard and red had a few moments, especially early in the week, or late in the week, depending on how well the kids treated me. However, this cycle did not last.

When we get closer to the end of the school year, and I become way more busy and worn out, Mr. Red band starts hogging all the attention! I feel just horrible! So bad! End of the world kinda' pain!

It's to be expected. Teachers get tired, students get tired, administrators get tired. And it affects everyone! And because I'm already naturally a step ahead of most people in the world of pain and suffering, It seems to affect me more.

In the beginning it was *"Oh, Jed is red today!"* But, after I wear it every day for almost a month, it starts to become less of a huge announcement. Don't get me wrong, my team still notices my red days and still understands that I may not be functioning at 100%, but I feel the true meaning of the "red day" has worn off.

Most everyone who has a chronic illness knows this feeling. When you're sick so often people just begin to ignore you. Nothing against them. I think it is a very natural human response. People just accept something as normal and move on.

It's like when I spent four years commuting a 90 miles round trip to St. Louis and back every day. At first it sucked, then I just got used to it and it didn't feel like I was driving that much. I just got used to it. We all do this with our own conditions. We eventually just get used to it. I've hurt every day of my life for 30 years. And for a while, I didn't think anything was wrong. Pain became a part of life and I forgot what life without pain was.

If I wore my green band every day and then suddenly went red, people would notice. When I wear my red band every day, people stop noticing.

For the people in my life, RED becomes normal. Just like for us, RED becomes normal. We don't always make a big deal out of it, and neither do they.

When I'm feeling bad I seclude myself to an empty conference room. At first people would walk in and say *"Oops, Jed is in his cave again!"* Now that I have sat in this room, for break and lunch, every day the same people no longer say anything when they walk in. They do, however, make a comment when they spot me in the lunchroom now. I broke away from normal.

As chronic illness advocates, we need to avoid falling into the "normal zone." Yes, it is comfortable there, people stop asking questions, and you are allowed to suffer in silence, (which is sometimes nice). But, if we want to have any chance of getting our diagnoses noticed, we need to break peoples' trances and break from the normal. We need to clash! Not like in a military sense, but more in a Tim Gunn, *"This isn't working, stripes and polka dots don't go together"* sense.

We need to find new ways to get noticed! Try new things! Make more noise, less noise, or at least a different noise. If you sit in the corner crying every day, after a while, people will just walk past you. If what you're doing isn't working, come up with a new plan, or get a louder voice.

I know, it sucks.

However, and this is my final point, when your advocacy starts to suck, the best thing you can do is get some help. If you don't have the spoons to get louder, combine your voices! A few quiet people still make more noise than one loud person for half the cost.

Go online and find people just like you who not only will notice you, but have the experience to build you up when you are feeling down.

Don't suffer in silence because others stop listening. Get noticed again and make them listen.

Don't let your red band become a cloak of invisibility.

Stacey Buchanan

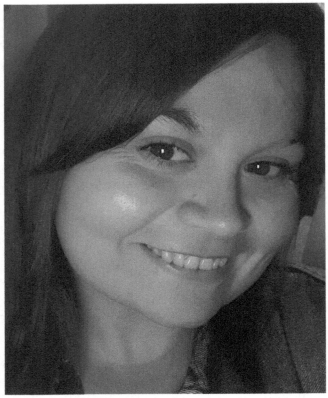

"My illness may sometimes be invisible, but I am not."

When first asked to contribute a short story to this amazing book, I had many ideas in my head about what I'd write about. Perhaps my diagnosis and the changes it made to my life. My operations, my treatments, my long list of medications and failed treatments that finally led to ones that made a difference. I even considered delving into the depression I experience, that inevitably comes with living daily with chronic pain.

I even contemplated sharing my positive experiences of what I feel has come from my diagnosis. But today I again encountered one of those many incidents we disabled and chronically ill inevitably experience. That frustrating occurrence of feeling invisible.

First off, I'm going to briefly explain my disability. I was diagnosed with juvenile arthritis just after my 10th birthday. I had endured the pain and fatigue for well over a year, but JIA is one of those things doctors do not automatically jump to when presented with a child experiencing pain. I was unfortunately not one of the lucky few that went into remission with JIA and, by the time I was 18, it was in all my joints. They say in life practice makes perfect but with JIA there's no preparation, nor getting used to it. You learn to live with it the best you can. No two days are the same. No two people have the exact same experiences like many chronic illnesses. JIA is a very lonely existence.

You can be surrounded by love and support. You can talk to other sufferers but in the end it's you. No one else truly can understand each day what you have. Each experience you have, each pain you endure . We learn to do things the best we can. We learn to adapt. We are strong people. We don't really have a choice to be or we will drown. Which is why when people talk like we aren't there, talk down to us, it makes all our daily fights feel wasted. I fight my body every day. I fight my mind every day. The last thing I want to do is fight a stranger to be heard.

When I am using my wheelchair, I have found people seem to associate that as I am deaf, I am stupid I cant do things for my self. Since childhood and early teen years I've experienced many moments of people talking about me, around me, like my disability has somehow removed my ability to talk, to hear and to understand. Many conversations were questions about me and were asked to the person I was with. Luckily my friend or family member would say- *"ask her not me it's not about me"* but not a lot of people have a family that takes that cue, they will answer for them.

We of course need support but support and taking over completely seems to be a fine line that most people don't see. We have extra hurdles to overcome than you but we are no different, we have the same fundamental wants and needs. We want relationships, some of us want children, we want stability, we want love and happiness. We want our independence but most of all we just want to be treated with kindness, compassion and most of all respect.

I'm extremely grateful for my family and friends and my whole support system. They have helped me be me, maintain my self worth, my independence and have never questioned my own thoughts or feelings on things, especially with my JIA journey. Living with a chronic illness unfortunately means giving up a lot of control. Life can be very unpredictable, but with a chronic illness unpredictable is our normal. So to me, getting to maintain my independence makes my life experiences that more meaningful.

Carmen Stokley

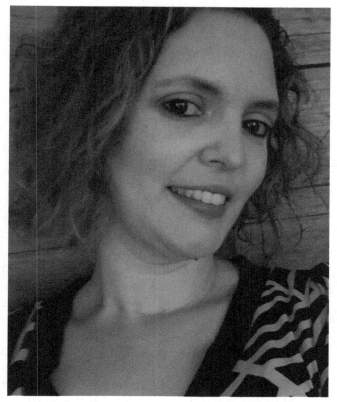

"Don't let your arthritis define you. Rather, let it be a small part of who you are."

One of my first memories is going to the doctor for my dislocated hip. I was four going on five years old. I was walking funny and my leg just hurt for no reason at all. My mama questioned me for a while: *"did I fall, did one of my siblings kick me?"* The answer was always no. I even tried to hide it for a few days, afraid of what my punishment would be! My memories are fuzzy now as so many years have gone by, but I do remember having to walk in just a shirt and panties, in a room full of adults, toward a man I barely knew, while another videoed me and my weird walk. It was awkward and set me up for a lifetime of being guarded and uneasy toward all males.

To this day, I have a difficult time talking to men, especially if they have any authority over me. I had to have fluid drawn from that hip and, while I don't remember the procedure, I bear the scar as proof it happened. Ultrasound, x-rays, and MRIs became second nature to me. I loved going to Cook Children's Hospital in Fort Worth for one reason. It was just me and my mom and she took me out to eat after every appointment, a treat for a poor kid from the projects with four other brothers and sisters.

Fast forward to elementary school. I was in the fourth grade when my doctors decided I no longer needed to participate in PE. I was secluded to the classroom with a book and told to "keep quiet," while the others played and had fun. While it instilled in me my lifetime love of reading, it was humiliating at first and made me "that weird girl." I didn't make friends easily after that and depression hit hard that year and the next.

Let's fast forward again to high school. In the 10th grade, I had to have hand surgery for a ganglion cyst on my left hand, my dominant hand. I was already awkward and shy around men, so when my biology teacher asked me the day after surgery what happened (I had a ginormous cast I couldn't hide, no matter what I tried), I had to tell the whole class that I have rheumatoid arthritis and had to have surgery so i could write without pain. I was once again humiliated by a man in front of a crowd, this time my peers.

Then there was the time I wanted to play softball in 11th grade. I bought a glove and a ball and started practicing my pitching with my older brother. I got quite good too, but the dreaded physical came and I was told I could not participate due to low cartilage in my left arm. Devastation reigns again. I just wanted to be a normal girl!!

Now, as a woman of 38, I look back and see how my disease shaped who I am as a person for so very long. At 18 it was confirmed that I carried the disease into adulthood and would need to continue treatment. I put my foot down and said no more shots, no more pills, no more injections, and by God no more surgeries!! I went 20 years on Tylenol and pain tolerance alone. By doing so I caused more damage than good. I have been seeing a wonderful rheumatologist now for the past four months and I am feeling better. The depression comes and goes, so I decided to seek help for that too, as I am obviously never going to be "well." If you get anything from my story, know that juvenile rheumatoid arthritis can shape a child's future in so many ways. Educate, and encourage your children so they don't get as easily discouraged and depressed as I did.

Grayson Schultz

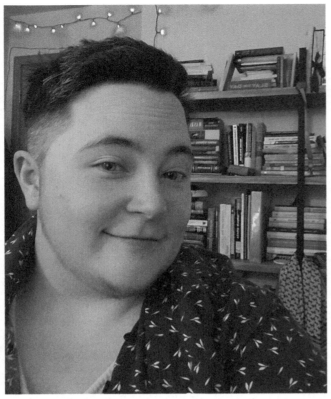

"It took 27 years of having arthritis to have someone outside of healthcare respond to my health shit in the way I needed them to - the way I deserve. Instead of advice or jumping to conclusions or cure evangelism, they were just there with me in that moment."

Note from author: The pieces in italics are snippets from my journal.

One November day, things in my body switched forever. Instead of a robust and healthy immune system, my innate immune system went haywire. I had fevers daily, one time even reaching 106 degrees, which also caused convulsions. A blotchy salmon-colored rash would cover my body at night, being invisible by the morning in the doctor's office. I began losing weight and energy, transforming from a bubbly and precocious five-year-old to a tired one. I began to relate far more to my great-grandmother (who has multiple sclerosis) than to kids my age.

After finding no answers to allergies, my family doctor and his consulting physicians brought leukemia into the mix. I was so ill that they thought I'd die within six weeks.

Thankfully, they were wrong and we proved it. My family spent nights in the University of Oregon libraries, digging for medical conditions that matched my symptoms until we found the answer. Doctors were amazed they could tell that I had systemic juvenile idiopathic arthritis (SJIA) from my labs. We know, though, that it is a diagnosis of exclusion.

As arthritis coursed through my body, causing irreversible damage, my mother worked her own brand of magic on the outside. I became isolated, unable to see health care providers. Then, she pulled me out of school with the notion of homeschooling me. That quickly turned into me educating myself, unfortunately.

Through it all, Mother would remind me that it would be hard to find someone to love me, that I'd never find a partner who treated me the way she did. Likely spurred by *her* mother's comments, she was adamant that I'd be living with her until the day one of us died.

Like any other abusive relationship, she used a weakness she saw as a way to obtain and maintain total control over my life.

I haven't spoken to Mother in eight years. The freedom that distance has brought is something that's hard to put into words. And yet, that isn't the only relationship that I've lost in part due to my arthritis.

My ex-husband and I were a decent match on the outside - similar levels of humor, really smart kids, and both dealing with depression. Early in our relationship, before he understood the severity of my health issues, he told me *"You aren't special. Everyone has pain."* Little did he know how often that saying popped into my head.

I was adamant that our relationship wouldn't fail, that we would beat the odds on divorce with arthritis. He struggled with his parents' divorce. My family background certainly didn't lead to a lot of speaking up. So, we both continued to avoid conflict, until divorce seeped in.

Being someone who does sex ed and helps people with relationships, I felt like a fraud. I tried to bring in communication techniques and help him get assistance in sharing his feelings. Between my health issues and discovering my gender, though, he assured me that things weren't salvageable.

It felt like my whole world was falling apart. I could hear my mother in my head:

"No one is going to love you, honey - not like I do."

I leaned into my queerness and my transness. In January 2020, I started testosterone, began using a new first name, and started to dress more masculinely. Truly, I began to lean into who I was, spending time working on myself and not working on others as much.

In the fall of 2020, I matched with someone on a dating app. Really, I was looking for someone to connect with in a way that embraced the sides of me I had found. The world thankfully had other plans. I wasn't planning on it being a long-term thing by any means. I mean, they lived in Ohio and I was in Wisconsin. How long-term could this get?

Not even a month later, we began to plan a cabin getaway inspired by a short story I wrote at their request. I pulled together spreadsheets for planning that included sharing emergency health information and talking more about my health issues. I waited until we were on video calls or in-person to go into details.

For the first time, I felt heard.

I didn't know when or how, but I knew the second that I got into my car to drive back to Wisconsin that I'd build a life with this amazing human.

I am very full of love, stability, assuredness, self-loving, eagerness, present, seen, authentic, validated, connected, brave, desirable, and most of all worthy. I have to explore that. If I got to spend the rest of my life with them? It'd be amazing.

I visited again after a few weeks, this time due to their father's passing. Even though it was for negative reasons, the love and support that I was given was incredible. Being able to meet my partner's mom and support her during such a tough time really meant a lot to me.

Two months later, I was back in Ohio again for my partner's birthday. I got to meet close cousins and have some vital conversation.

While in Ohio, I had a conversation with Grav about my arthritis - the ways it shows up and how it can be fatal. It's something that I've struggled with in part because it feels like people really don't listen.

In 2007, when I met my ex-husband, I had to write these things out. I was in college and not emotionally developed enough to have these conversations verbally. He acted like many things I dealt with were things all people experienced. It felt like I had to scream to be heard in that relationship, that I wasn't taken seriously about anything.

Leaving that marriage and getting on testosterone helped me find myself again. My sister says that I'm the most 'me' I've been in ages, and she's not wrong.

Talking about these issues with McGravin in person...was so different. They listened. They asked questions.

It took 27 years of having arthritis to have someone outside of healthcare respond to my health shit in the way I needed them to - the way I deserve. Instead of advice or jumping to conclusions or cure evangelism, they were just there with me in that moment.

Still, being long-distance was hard. I felt like I was counting down the seconds until I saw them again, spending more time hanging out on video chat with them than doing stuff in the 'real world.' The plus, of course, is that this happened during the pandemic.

In the summer of 2021, we went on a trip as a family back to the Adirondacks town where Grav's mom grew up. When we hiked, how much space they gave me still floors me. There was no judgment for needing to rest, even if it was every five minutes.

I worried about how my upcoming top surgery - a surgery to masculinize my chest - would go. While I am historically not great at relying on others or asking for help, they were coming up to help and be there for me during recovery. Still, I was worried about them seeing first-hand what it's like when I'm off my arthritis medications for weeks at a time. Part of me feared that they would see something that screamed, *"Run! Get out while you still can!"*

In the end, I'm glad Grav was around because I almost died. One of my comorbidities hit hard during intubation and sent my body into crisis. My providers were prepared and able to get things under control enough to complete the surgery, but I was told I should avoid future surgeries if at all possible. It wasn't exactly news that I was happy to wake up to, but having a flat chest made it all worth it.

After an unplanned overnight in the hospital, my knight in shining armor helped me get dressed and took me home. For the next five days, they were constantly by my side to help me bathe, change my surgical dressings, and empty drainage tubes.

In mid-August, Grav visited again - this time to help me move to Ohio. It's May of 2022 as I write this, and I'm still floored that I've spent every single day with them since then.

Has every day been perfect? No. Have we disagreed on things? Absolutely. Have we 'fought'? I wouldn't say so. This time, though, it isn't because I think conflict or disagreement is bad. It's because I know these things are small and often inconsequential.

Differences of opinion are so tiny when they're handled with emotional maturity, or when people aren't keeping score.

My arthritis? We view it the way I've always recommended to others - as something we have to deal with together. It's made so much difference in how we approach each other.

As Maren Morris sings, *"When the bones are good, the rest don't matter"*

Emma Cross

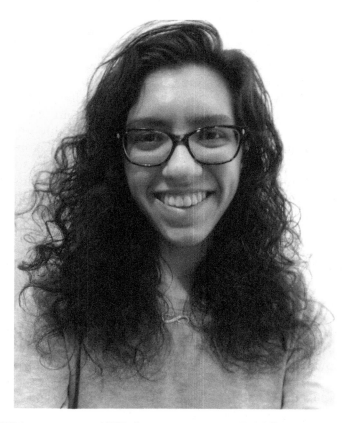

"It can still be a good life even with challenges and pain."

Everyone talks about the amazing experiences you'll have in your twenties. Your college years, your twenties, are supposed to be filled with exciting new experiences, taking risks, and having fun! Getting diagnosed with rheumatoid arthritis during my first year of college was not part of the plan. RA definitely was not the fun new experience I had been hoping for when I headed off to college. My chronic illness became a hidden burden. I didn't know who to tell, how to tell them, or if I even wanted anyone to know. When I did share my diagnosis with others, I significantly downplayed the impact it had on my body and my life. After I got sick just a few months before my 20th birthday, my arthritis symptoms only got worse. My mobility became more limited and I found myself frequently walking with a limp because of

my stiff, swollen knees. I did my best to hide this from people, not wanting them to think less of me. I was especially worried that my boyfriend's parents would attempt to dissuade their son from dating me - after all, who wants their healthy child to have to carry the burden of a disabled partner? Even though they'd given no indication that they felt this way, I found myself downplaying and lying about my arthritis.

That summer, my sister got married. In the weeks leading up to the wedding, my movement became even more limited as my arthritis went unchecked without proper medications. I continued to flare in my hands, knees, and feet. I was supposed to be a bridesmaid but I was not sure if I would even be able to walk down the aisle that day. I remember my sister's wedding as a beautiful and happy event. But behind those positive memories, there are also memories of my pain. I walked down the aisle, but I couldn't dance at the reception. At the end of the night, I needed others to help me walk. I crawled up the stairs of my home. It was not the first time my arthritis would interfere with my life (and it certainly would not be the last), but I had never witnessed before how impactful my condition could be.

Medication gave me my body back. I had pushed off trying certain medications because of fears I had, not only about the side effects on my body, but also the side effects on my social life. What would people think of me having to take all these medications? Those months showed me though, that whether I took medication or not, my RA would impact my social life. Trying a new medication plan with my rheumatologist was an attempt to take my life back.

The medication helped, however, rheumatoid arthritis is a chronic condition. Instead of leaving all those challenges in the past, I continue to carry the emotional weight. What if I have a flare-up again during another significant life event? Will I have to miss my graduation? What if I cannot walk down the aisle at my own wedding? Not only is the arthritis chronic, but so is the anxiety that comes with it. My arthritis has made me miss out on a lot of events that are "supposed to be" part of the young adult experience. Will I have to miss out on even more? My arthritis is not going away and it is not going to become predictable either. I am left with uncertainty about my future, never knowing if I will feel well enough to participate in life. Making plans does not seem to make much sense when you know the plan will have to change. This is all incredibly frustrating. I am still trying to process my grief and anger. But, despite the negative feelings I'm still grappling with, I recognize that my rheumatoid arthritis is not always stealing my joy, but is in many ways a catalyst for good changes.

My RA limits me, but that makes me appreciate even more when I can go out and live the typical 20-something year old life. My RA has pushed me to find community in new places such as online spaces for individuals with chronic illness. I have learned that my time and energy are valuable; I have to be more discerning now with how I spend that time and energy, but in many ways that's a good thing. I am choosing to be an advocate for myself. I need to prioritize myself (and particularly my health), instead of being a people pleaser. Having RA has forced me to become a better communicator in regards to my health needs. It has been two years since that wedding and while I was afraid and ashamed for others to see me struggling then, I am much more up-front with others about my limitations now. It has been invaluable to find others that understand and who don't mind canceling a night out to have a chill, comfortable night in instead. It is okay to ask for help and accommodations.

I'm still struggling with the "what if" questions. I also often still feel jealousy for those who do not experience the social limitations which are imposed on me by my health. I do not have my social life figured out and my rheumatoid arthritis makes that really difficult at times. However, the challenges I face push me to be creative, help me to find the people that really care about and understand me, to prioritize and advocate for myself, and to recognize the struggles others are facing. I am much more likely now to recognize how certain places may be physically inaccessible to people, or why someone may not be able to attend a social event. Ultimately, the challenges I've faced and continue to face due to my arthritis, have helped me learn how to have more compassion for others and for myself. Maybe I won't have the typical twenties experience, but I will continue to try my best to take things one day at a time and enjoy being social in whatever ways my body will allow each day. I can be angry sometimes that my young adult experience is not the typical one (and it's okay to be angry or sad about it), but it can still be a good life even with times of challenge and pain that are sure to come.

Suruthi Gnanenthiran

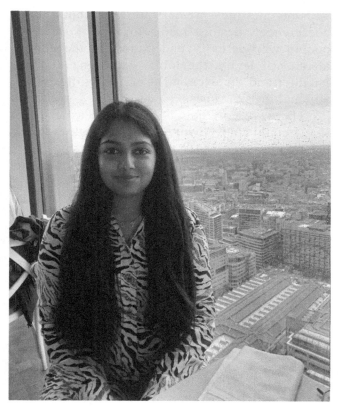

"Life with arthritis can suck sometimes, but you may be able to do something that makes it suck just a little bit less!"

Being diagnosed with arthritis (specifically JIA) as a young child, was never going to do wonders for my social calendar, but growing older, I realize just how taxing it can be. I always say having a chronic illness is like a full-time admin job - between chasing up appointments and blood test results, booking scans and ordering prescriptions, it is hard work! However, I decided I no longer want it to derail my social life so here are the stories of how I sometimes achieve the balance... and how sometimes it doesn't go to plan.

Let's start with appointments. I have recently made a habit of making plans before afternoon appointments or plans much later in the evening. For the most part, it is a good idea in theory where I either get to have fun before or have something to look forward to after. Whichever one it is, I will always get a 'treat myself' Starbucks at the hospital. The first time I tried making dinner plans after an appointment, I started to see the cracks in my plan. I had a birthday dinner to go to about 3 ½ hours after my appointment, and it was only a 20 minute walk away so I thought it would be fine, and even thought I may have time to go home and relax for a bit before dinner. What I still sometimes forget is that hospital appointments, much like chronic illnesses, can be really quite unpredictable. I started stressing a bit when I still hadn't been called in an hour after the appointment time, but once I was in with the consultants, it was all smooth sailing. They told me my eyes were good, my uveitis was dormant and just carry on with the same eye drops. With two hours till dinner, I was so excited! Yet as we discuss next appointment dates and so on, they ask me to quickly pop up for a blood test and stop by the hospital pharmacy to collect more eye drops. My excitement quickly faded as I joined the blood test queue with 20 people ahead. Even when it was my turn, my shy veins that refused to reveal themselves made my blood test feel like forever (okay fine it was only five minutes). The time was now half an hour to dinner and it was time to start walking over. Only as I am almost there with the restaurant in sight do I realize... I never got my prescription. Moral of this story is to stick to plans before appointments, or give yourself plenty of hours when making plans after.

Next, infusions! My treatment consists of a two hour infusion every month which makes me feel quite tired so I usually just watch tv or read in bed for the rest of the day. These are my favorite hobbies anyway, but when the weather is nice and everyone's out having fun, sometimes I feel a bit left out. I know better than to make plans to meet friends on infusion day because I will just be too knackered to even leave the house. However, adult life means you often have friends spread across the country, sometimes even dotted all around the world, and catch ups with them mostly happen on Facetime. I love to schedule a call with a friend in the early evening, which gives me time to have a nap and some food after my infusion. It makes it a lot less lonely and makes me better at keeping in touch with my friends who live far away. You get to still socialize but without leaving the house, and still be in bed by 9 p.m. I call that a win in my books.

These may seem like the most simple suggestions but I spent a long time not doing these things, and adding these plans in around appointments and infusions has been so refreshing for my mental health and helped me cope a lot better. Life with arthritis can suck sometimes, but you may be able to do something that makes it suck just a little bit less!

Issadora Saeteng

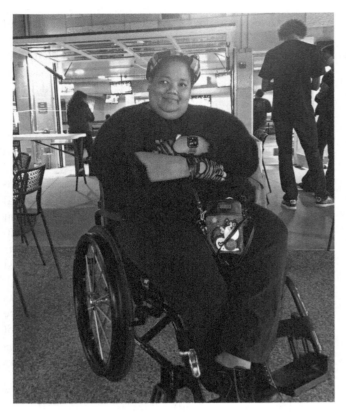

"When your universe and parallel universe go on 'A Real Trip' together."

CC (alias) and I had participated in a few of these conventions in prior years and the enjoyment was indescribable. Just being around hundreds of families, kids, teens, and young adults who are part of your own juvenile arthritis tribe!

The words, conference and conventions aren't typically synonymous with fun, excitement and a longing for another year to come around quickly!

Our friend, RR (alias) had never gone to a AJAO convention until this time where we all were able to go. She admitted that prior to these conventions. CC and I would chatter excitedly about them and show pictures trying to transmit the feelings that really can't come out of a few still photos. RR, after having gone with us, became indoctrinated into AJAO conference feelings. These don't come from the conference sessions at all.

One of the greatest things about these conferences, besides just being around loads of people who actually understand, is the endless amount of levity, the looks that bring knowing laughter and the excitement of seeing old friends and making new ones.

There are a plethora of stories and experiences that I could share involving love, laughter, tears, grief and inspiration.

Yet, out of seemingly infinite choices, after living with JIA for most of my life, the following kept moving to the forefront as a common theme but a different perspective.

Us three young ladies checked in the hotel early in the morning, quite a few hours before the welcome event began. A large banner with 'The Arthritis Foundation' in big bold letters and the insignia at that time, hung from the entryway to the conference areas.

Since we were there early, we decided to take a trip to the mall using the hotel's complimentary service. A young, rather handsome guy was our driver. He was so friendly with hardly veiled flirting which we stoked in kind. He readily gave us his name and number to personally request his shuttle.

We were excited and toured for a while enjoying the startling green hue that the plants, trees and bushes displayed. At one point, I started chuckling about how much it must be obvious that we are tourists because the light is green for us to cross, yet the 3 of us are standing, with our backs to the street, around this bush, touching and staring and attempting to capture the situation with the, not stellar, 'throw away' cameras frequently used back then.

We called our cute driver for the return and he was there so quickly, with a big flirty smile, and asked about our adventures which we relayed.

Back at the hotel, as he's sliding open the van door, he says, *'well ladies, please call me for rides wherever you want, especially because this place is going to be SO BORING because a lot of OLD PEOPLE are coming for The Arthritis Foundation convention,''* with a rolling eyeball and tone of dismay...definitely uncool was transmitting from his body. Us three ladies busted a gut with uproarious laughter ever so heartily as he looked surprised and confused.

Finally, one of us could control our giggles long enough to tell him... 'mmmm. WE have arthritis and are here for the conference (deeper looks of confusion), as it's for families and young adults with juvenile arthritis. No old people here!' We laughed even harder as he was blushing with embarrassment.

Despite this typically being a tiresome line, heard way too frequently in our daily lives, it was instead, refreshing and funny together as JA friends, part of our greater tribe converging upon this place.

It was a real trip' for him more than for us.

We didn't see him at all over the three day convention! He was probably too busy transporting all of us 'boring old people"

A real trip!

Taylor Van Emmerik

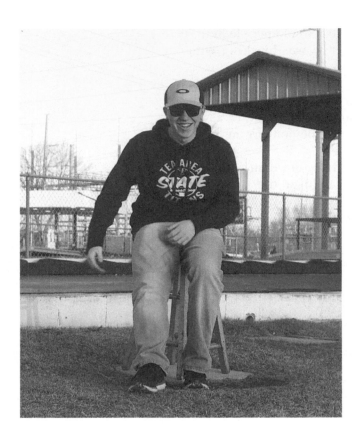

"Everyone has a story to tell, and each story- no matter how small- can make a huge difference."

Standing on my school's gym floor felt like an eternity as I waited for students to file into their seats, so I could share my story of living with arthritis. The line seemed to go on forever, and with each new person coming into the gym, I felt time start to get slower and slower. My nerves started to grow, and they brought pain along with them. The piece of paper in front of me that I had already edited over 15 times, now seemed futile.

"What should I talk about?" I asked myself.

This would be the first time some of these people have ever heard of arthritis. How could I do justice for all the arthritis warriors out there? I could talk about having to travel over four hours just to see a pediatric rheumatologist who could point at me and say, *"Aha, you have polyarticular juvenile idiopathic arthritis!"* Wait, what about the three doctors I saw before that who couldn't tell me what was wrong with me? Or how about going to school for the next couple of weeks and trying to explain to my friends why I had to sit out from activities and wear a boot, when even I didn't have a clue what was going on?

Should I talk about the pain?

Wow, how creative!

Should I talk about the swelling and my loss of grip strength?

Wow, are you really going to bring up that your ankle was the size of a water balloon again, or how you couldn't close your hands enough to get dressed?

Should I talk about the restless nights lying in bed because no matter what I do the pain seems too unbearable? Should I talk about the countless medications I found myself all of sudden having to take? Or the constant threat of having things become worse if we didn't get it under control? Or how about the time I made it into remission, just to discover that my arthritis had come back and I now had it in nearly double the number of joints as before. That should about cover it right?

Wait, what about the over 300,000 other kids, in the United States alone, who have similar stories to mine? Or the over 54 million adults in the United States suffering from arthritis, (at the time), with their own stories to tell. No, no... That hardly seems adequate to explain arthritis.

Then I was reminded of something I had heard at camp many times before, *"Everyone has a story to tell, and each story- no matter how small- can make a huge difference."* I had been given a unique opportunity to bring awareness to a disease in which few people understand. Not only this, but I had been given a unique perspective as someone experiencing it first hand. I may not have had arthritis since I was born. I may not be adhered to a wheelchair because of it. I may not have to do injections every week, but none of that means I don't know the pain of arthritis. The pain, the swelling, the limitations, the unspoken side effects of being someone living with arthritis all apply to me. This isn't just about me. It's about letting people know what's going on with me and thousands of others.

All of a sudden, my principal came over to me, patted me on the shoulders, and asked *"Are you ready? It's go time!"*

I looked over at him, nodded, and walked to the center of the gym: *"One day in June of 2013, my life changed forever. Hi, my name is Taylor Van Emmerik and I am an arthritis warrior. This is my story..."*

Note From Taylor: *One part of arthritis, that just comes with the territory, is telling others about how you feel. You tell your doctors your pain level for the day. You warn your teachers and set up plans preparing for the worst. You have to explain to your friends why you aren't able to hangout. It's hard. It's not easy to tell people about your flaws. It's EXHAUSTING. It's tiring to have to repeatedly explain what is going on, but yet, we have to do it. It's probably not what you signed up for when you signed up for this arthritis thing (haha as if anyone would willingly sign up for this). Nevertheless, it's one of the most important things you can do for all the people who will eventually need to be welcomed into the community. You may feel your story isn't worth spreading, you may think you can't do it, but you have been given a unique opportunity in this world to bring light to a disability that people only think the elderly get. And, who knows, you may even give encouragement to someone fighting alongside you. My wish for you is that you find your voice, whether big or small and see where it takes you.*

Anonymous

"I loved her little hand gripping my finger and having my first skin-to-skin with her in the NICU. From this experience, I learned that I am a health warrior. I'm a rheumatoid arthritis warrior, fibromyalgia warrior, celiac disease warrior, and most importantly, a bad-ass mama, wife, and person with invisible or non-apparent disabilities."

Dear Dr.,

As your colleague may have shared, I had a traumatic labor and delivery experience. I had a preterm premature rupture of the membranes, and was considered a high-risk pregnancy due to my rheumatoid arthritis. My water broke in my bed during week 32, and the goal was to keep me pregnant until week 34. During my emergency hospital stay, I experienced lots of loneliness, trying to keep myself busy because my husband needed to continue teaching, so he could utilize his sick time once our daughter was born. I was stressed and anxious that my daughter and I would be okay.

During that time, I would hear all the hospital alarms and codes, the rush of the hospital staff getting a laboring mother to the operating room, and so much more. I started to count the number of times I heard a baby cry, knowing that another baby was born, and I recall hearing a natural delivery. Hearing the babies cry was the only thing that kept my mood up when I was alone and my nurses could not keep me company. When the nurse told me that the scream I heard was from a natural delivery, I laughed, "I'm glad I am going to get an epidural." Some of the nurses were sweet and tried to accompany me to ease the stress of my labor experience throughout the days leading up to my daughter's birth, since my husband was at work and I could only have one labor coach due to the pandemic.

February 24th was the day. Within the remaining six to seven hours of the labor process, I went from zero centimeters dilated to completely dilated. I could not pinpoint some of my psychological triggers until I went through the labor and delivery process. My nurse, assigned to me during those last hours leading up to my daughter's birth, was very dismissive and did not take my concerns seriously. She told me there was nothing they could do for my pain and would not accommodate me when I asked if I could rest on my side, and have the belly monitor moved, like how the other nurses accommodated me. She tightened it so tight that I remember having indentations on my stomach. I suffered unbearable pain during that time because the nurse forced me to remain on my back, creating excruciating pain in my back and right hip through the contractions, so they could make sure my daughter was doing okay.

My labor plan was to have an epidural, and I lost the opportunity to have that happen. I recall the nurse coming into my room at one point, after they had already administered morphine, asking how I was feeling. I remember telling her that I had terrible contractions, even with the morphine. I had a lot of emotional pain too, because every time I had severe contractions, the right side of my back and hip would hurt badly, which is the same side that I injured at my previous job and I currently have a lawsuit against them. I knew I had to utter the word lawsuit for the nurse to take me seriously. I have always heard how women of color and invisible disabilities like mine are treated poorly in the medical system. I now fully believe it.

After I uttered the word lawsuit within a minute or less, I remember the doctor and my nurse rushing back into my room. I remember the doctor saying that she didn't want to do this, but she had to do a digit check to see how much I dilated. She didn't want to risk my child or me getting an infection, but she needed to see if I had dilated since the previous doctor checked earlier in the evening. So she checked, and I was 10 centimeters dilated. My husband shared that I was frothing blood as the doctor pulled her hands out and at that moment, he knew it was about to happen. I remember the doctor saying we were having a baby today, and I was terrified about having a premature baby.

I immediately remember a rush of people coming into my room prepping for the delivery team, the NICU team, L&D team, anesthesiologist technician, and I think a respiratory therapist. I recall seeing all the tools on the table for the epidural, which freaked me out even more. So many tools! I remember a bright blue bag being placed under me to catch all the fluids and blood during my delivery process. I remember them putting a hair net on me and an oxygen mask on my face, and my husband stroking my head to comfort me before the process started.

As I went through each bad contraction, my right leg would shake uncontrollably, and I was in excruciating pain in my right back and hip; I recall the pain wrapping around my right side to my belly button. The shaking only happened on the right side of my back, hip, and leg. As this all happened, I had flashbacks of my fall and traumatic encounters at my previous employer. I was so mad that during my labor process, these flashbacks were popping up during one of the most pivotal times of my life. I was in pain, hurting, and angry. While I had all these internal emotions, I appeared calmer on the outside while still in normal delivery pain.

After one of these contractions and while we were all waiting for the anesthesiologist to come, I looked at my L&D doctor and said, *"I cannot safely sit through an epidural."* I remember she said, *"Okay, we got this, I'm going to coach you through the whole process, and we're going to get through this."* I remember pushing for roughly thirty minutes, and my husband and the nurses, including the dismissive nurse, had to be my

stirrups since I was in a regular hospital bed, not a labor and delivery bed. I remember they told me to push by pushing my pelvis forward and pulling my legs towards my chest. I remember the pain being so bad through each contraction that I was driving my legs against them instead of pulling my legs. I was doing that because I had the worst pain in my right back, hip, and right side of my stomach. I eventually realized that she would only come out if I pulled my legs towards me. I think I did one or two pushes correctly before she finally burst out, and I remember feeling my vagina tear.

I was relieved that she was out, but I was so sad and shocked that I mainly thought about my old job. I've done a lot of reflecting since I delivered. When I was in the hospital, I texted my therapist, letting her know I was in preterm labor. She connected with me again when I was in the hospital to see how I was doing. I told her that my daughter was born and that I would like to see her sooner than we initially had planned to meet. I was discharged on February 26th and had a virtual therapy appointment that Monday. I cried the entire session. That was the first time that I cried throughout a whole therapy session. I knew I was in a bad state when she said, *"Would you like to meet with me on Thursday as well? I can tell you have a lot that you are processing."*

I did not have the labor and delivery experience that I wanted. People say hope for the best and expect the worst; I had terrible labor and delivery. However, seeing my daughter for the first time was like the rainbow at the end of my storm. Although she had numerous wires attached to her, due to being a preemie in the NICU, I knew they were essential to her growth and development. I loved being reconnected with her and seeing her for the first time. I loved her little hand gripping my finger and having my first skin-to-skin with her in the NICU. From this experience, I learned that I am a health warrior. I'm a rheumatoid arthritis warrior, fibromyalgia warrior, celiac disease warrior, and most importantly, a bad-ass mama, wife, and person with invisible or non-apparent disabilities.

Samantha Johnson

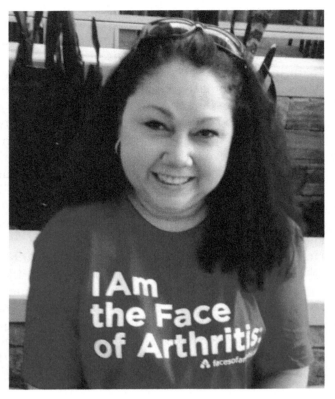

"Find your people!"

It was the year 2000. I was in my senior year at Arizona State University with my BA Degree in Women's Studies. My area of concentration was, "Women with Disabilities." Part of my curriculum included completing an internship. With my area of concentration being a new concept, I was offered a unique opportunity. I was approved to complete my internship by the Department Head, which consisted of bringing the first ever, "Women with Disabilities" conference," to the College. I oversaw all the aspects of putting the conference together, under the management of the internship professor. I worked on the entire organization of the conference; where, when, how, all the accommodation and technology needed. Also, I was required to bring together a panel of student speakers with disabilities. It was in this process that I met two different young women that shared my disability.

The three of us were in different stages of JRA/RA. This was the very first time I had met anyone "like me," that looked like me and understood what I was going through trying to live with arthritis. This was "my tribe." It only took me 30 years to meet anyone like me. I went through a roller coaster of emotions of course. The day came to have our conference. One of the many questions that were asked of the students on the panel was asked of me. *"After you graduate, what kind of job will you get with this degree?"* I answered, *"Well, I will probably end up in Washington DC advocating for people with disabilities, because that is exactly what I do Not want to do."* Laughter filled the air.

Let me tell you, that is exactly what I did! I became an advocate for people with arthritis, especially people like me. I called it a "coming home." Where I decided to focus on arthritis as the specific disability I would advocate for. I went to the Arizona State Capital for an advocate day, planned with the Arthritis Foundation. And eventually I made it to Washington DC as an advocate for arthritis as well. But the most rewarding thing I did, after earning my degree in Women's Studies/Women with Disabilities, so far was to be afforded another opportunity in founding a non-profit organization called "Arthritis Introspective." It was solely based on the fact that as a person with arthritis, in the prime of their life, college age-working-and starting a family, being able to find support was lacking in the community. We wanted to meet our people. There was support for the children with arthritis and for the elderly with arthritis. But there was not any for the entire group of us in between.

So sometimes when there is nothing relatable available you must make it. We built it and they came. Our tribe!, "AI – Arthritis Introspective," has since dissipated into the universe. But it lasted 10 years. Many friendships were formed across the US. Other groups were formed from ours. The Internet is one of those avenues now. I found my tribe. I am an advocate, and I would not have it any other way.

SPIRITUALITY & FAITH

Stories

Isabella McCray

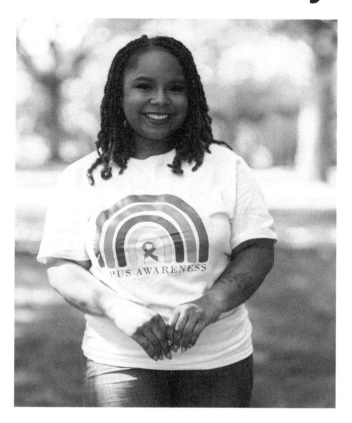

**"Despite my limitations, I developed patience
and discovered hope in the worst of situations.
Because battling a life-altering illness is a tough journey
and changing directions in life is not a bad decision."**

Seeing the words "no cure" left me questioning everything I thought I had figured out in life. When I was little, I went to preschool and my teacher used to always rub and massage my legs because my legs were always sore. Eventually, it became difficult to run and play, to climb stairs, and if I had exposure to sunlight/heat, I would break out in hives. I went to my pediatrician and she diagnosed me with growing pains. Years passed and it was time for my annual check up with my pediatrician. She saw visibly swollen glands and referred me to an ear nose and throat (ENT)

doctor. He discovered abnormalities in my blood labs and referred me to my present pediatric rheumatologist. I was diagnosed with lupus and rheumatoid arthritis in 2014. I was on many medications and for a while, I felt suffocated and lost. I recall searching what it was and reading about the symptoms. I experienced each of them. Joint pain, headaches, fatigue, butterfly rash, hair loss, etc. I was just 11 when I was diagnosed with lupus. I was a young child and I didn't know how to feel or how to accept my diagnosis. I also didn't know that my life would change forever. In the years following, I learned to manage my chronic illness that had no cure. I had a life-changing flare up in 2017 and I was homebound for seven months, and I was in and out of the hospital. I shared my diagnosis with my school peers, school staff and church members. Word got around in school and I was treated differently.

I looked different because of my treatments and my hair started to shed. In light of my insecurities and challenges, I decided to cut my hair. I was a victim of bullying. I was completely drained, hopeless, and depressed. All of these experiences happened because of one thing, lupus. I thought for a while I was not worthy of anything because who would want a "sick girl" in their life to be a burden on them. However, I didn't let the pain and suffering I endured break me. Instead, I started embracing the pain and turning it into strength and inspiration, and I only did that through my religious beliefs and faith in Jesus. The Bible was my #1 key to my healing. At my lowest he loved me, and I let that love, that grace, that adoration consume me.

I had to face unknown experiences, having hope and strength in Jesus and the mindset of coming out of these experiences even stronger. I became an advocate, not only for chronic illnesses, but also for my education as well. Being afforded the opportunity of encountering many doctors, and nurses on my various visits to the hospital inspired me to pursue and further my education in nursing to hopefully become a pediatric nurse.

I use my platform on social media to spread the word of God and talk about what it's like living and managing lupus. From my pre-teens, into my later teen years, I have needed to balance my health changes with my life changes. My spiritual growth in God is growing every day as my faith is rooted in His word. Despite my limitations, I developed patience and discovered hope in the worst of situations. Because battling a life-altering illness is a tough journey and changing directions in life is not a bad decision. It just allows you to change your story and experience the high and lows with an amazing support system. Throughout my journey, I learned to let go of the illusion that it could have been different and understand my purpose now. It's not every day I'm going to feel my best, but at the end of the day, I made it, and that itself is a victory. Know your limitations, enjoy life, take your medications, and be yourself, because an illness does not define who you are.

Ashley Davis

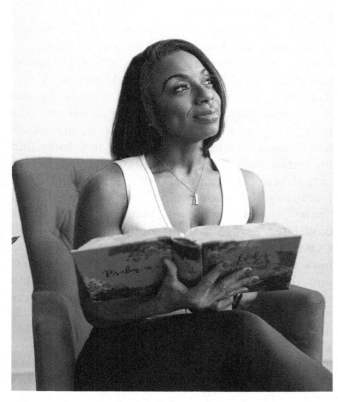

"I have RA, but RA does not have me. I choose faith over fear!"

I'm the master trainer, founder and coach at RA Warrior Fitness, where the mission is to empower women living with rheumatoid arthritis, and other chronic conditions, to improve their quality of life through FAITH, FOOD and FITNESS, while eliminating negative self-talk and strenuous exercise.

Faith is the number one pillar in the mission, because it is the foundation that pushes me through on the tough days of managing my RA. Having a positive mindset, and strong relationship with God, is the key to successful transformation and improving overall quality of life.

Exercising my spiritual muscles by reading the bible, prayer, meditation and repeating positive affirmations, have helped me to strengthen my mindset and overcome the daily challenges that come with RA. I coach on this topic in my program and it has benefited so many chronic illness warriors in their journey as well.

Having faith that God will continue to give me supernatural strength and resilience to rise above RA keeps me going each day. Not only having faith in God, but also having faith in myself that I can do all things through Christ who gives me strength. This goes back to mindset. The pain, discomfort and fatigue that comes with RA, can cause people to have limiting beliefs and feelings of depression and anxiety. Overall transformation is more than just food and exercise, it all starts with the mindset. When the mind and faith are strong, everything else will follow.

Gratitude is another way to exercise my mindset muscle and faith. There is always something to be thankful for regardless of what I'm feeling. Each time I have the opportunity to celebrate what my body can do is truly a blessing. There was a time when I would dwell on what I couldn't do and that made me feel inadequate. I felt like I wasn't "enough." I later learned that there are modifications to getting things done and I could still accomplish my goal. I don't take for granted that I can celebrate, and be grateful for what my body can do, instead of focusing on what it isn't able to do because of the physical limitations due to rheumatoid arthritis. When I learned how to modify a burpee, I couldn't stop!!! I AM ENOUGH! I AM CAPABLE! I AM A CONQUEROR! I AM A WARRIOR!

My favorite scripture is Jeremiah 29:11 which states, *"For I know the plans I have for you, declares the Lord. Plans to prosper you and not to harm you. Plans to give you hope and a future."* (The Bible, New International Version)

I'm thankful that God has allowed me to walk in my purpose, and turn my pain into purpose to help others in their faith walk, while living with RA. He will always give me hope and I'll forever have faith in Him and tell everyone just how GREAT He is!

Antoinette Atkinson

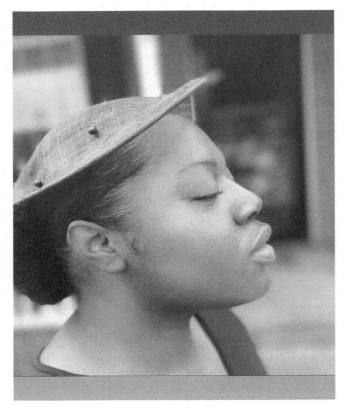

"Although rheumatoid arthritis is NOT pretty, life can still be beautiful. I am embracing 'new norms,' full of faith and comforted by peace that surpasses ALL understanding. RA and I aren't 'besties' BUT we do have a balance going. I guess you can call it 'Poetic Disharmony.'"

"Pre-Diagnosis"

I was back home from FMU, the last semester of my sophomore year had just ended.
"Mama, I feel this weird pricking pain in the top of my thumb."

This is the day that is etched into my memory as the first time I felt something "out of the norm," that had come out of nowhere. I was twenty years old. This was three years before an official diagnosis.

A few days after that I began feeling a strange pain within my knee. As a "heavier" individual, I automatically brushed it off as a "weight issue" and decided to just ice it and elevate it. A few days later I woke up in excruciating pain and discovered that my arm, below the elbow, was bent funny and I could not move it, my hands had become extremely sensitive and sore, and my wrist felt like they had developed severe carpal tunnel overnight...OUT OF NOWHERE. I actually thought my arm was broken. It even "hung" funny. I made an appointment, but a few days later, before that appointment, the pain had COMPLETELY DISAPPEARED. Everything was back to normal, except the pain within my wrists and the pain within my knees had noticeably increased. So we just brought a brace for my wrist, and I had begun using a single crutch to alleviate some of the pain and weight from that knee. At my appointment I had blood work done and, during her physical examination, she noticed that my hands had a bit of a tremor and I couldn't hold them still. We realized many years later that my inflammation markers had been slightly elevated back then. I guess it wasn't considered a "pressing" issue. Life went on but that experience was etched in my memory.

My junior year at FMU had begun. I was having quite an emotionally taxing time, and my course load was stressful and overwhelming me. Which I later found out is my MAIN flare trigger. Mid semester I was FINALLY assigned to this on campus apartment that was my DREAM spot. I got the news in the morning and by that night I had moved myself across campus by myself. I later found out that OVEREXERTION is also a MAIN flare trigger. A few days later I began noticing that one crutch wasn't alleviating enough of the pain and the weight seemed extra heavy. The bottoms of my feet had become very sore. I could only bear to stand/walk in thick slippers. My health continued to rapidly decline.

By the middle of my first junior semester, I now needed both crutches and I couldn't write, nor comb my hair. My mother had to move on campus to assist me, and eventually I had to make the heartbreaking decision to move back home and become a commuter, because my health had declined even more. I had become so ill that I barely left the bed. I was fatigued and weak. Around this same time my mother's health had also started to decline. I had to make the decision to completely medically withdraw. I was SO close to graduation and I had just gotten a taste of the life I had wanted for a long time. Only for me I had NO choice but to give it up.

Back at home my health had declined worse and I was now wheelchair bound. One day my mother noticed that I had lost a significant amount of weight, within a time span of two and a half months (about 70 pounds). That was alarming!! We were still trying natural remedies and holistic practices and we were planning to get me to a doctor for a check up. A few months later my mother passed away suddenly. The next month I made an appointment to get blood-work done.

"Day of Official Diagnosis"

"Darling, your blood is on fire! Not only do you have rheumatoid arthritis, you have it severely. We MUST start treatment immediately!"

There I sat. I had just turned twenty three years old the month before. After battling what I now know was RA ever since age twenty. This diagnosis had me bound to a wheelchair and bedridden. There I sat with no mother to console me and a life changing decision to make. My ankles were swollen with a thickness only open-back slippers could contain. My feet were overwhelmingly sore and sensitive. My knees were so inflamed that the heat was actually radiating, through the thick jean skirt my sisters had managed to slip me into. My knees and elbows were locked. My fingers stiff. I could not flex them at all. My muscles had wasted and I was left with little to no strength. My knees had become so weak and inflamed that I couldn't stand, not even WITH assistance. So walking hadn't been an option for the past year and a half.

"My blood is on fire?"

The doctor explained to me that the lab results showed extreme levels of inflammation with my rheumatoid factor actually being "unchartable." The average RA factor is not supposed to be higher than 14, yet somehow my RA factor

was BEYOND their systems max of 650. After many scans, tests, and x-rays we discovered that although everything about my case was extreme, AND my diagnosis classified as severe, I hadn't suffered any permanent damage. Thanks be to God!

I had spent the past three years undiagnosed and "untreated," just trying to fight "it" off naturally. Which may have worked, had my levels not been so extreme and my circumstances severe. Quite frankly, I was "juiced" out. I had digested SO much turmeric, ginger and raw beets during those years, so I decided to try what he advised along with the natural remedies.

"Okay. What do I need to do?"

The doctor then proceeded to educate me, advise me and prescribe me. I started my treatment that night.

Along with making a few dietary changes "cold turkey," I started noticing positive progress within that week. But because my inflammation markers were still high, a biologic was added to my treatment.

One month later my pain had decreased majorly and my locked joints had begun to move a bit. The next month some of my strength had returned. I was able to sit up and lift my legs... BY MYSELF!

The third month I was able to stand up briefly WITH ASSISTANCE!! That FOURTH MONTH though!!! I finally took my "first steps"! I was able to work my way back onto a roller with a seat attached (so that I could walk and be able to rest). Then came crutches and then a cane, and eventually I was able to walk UNASSISTED!!

"Present day"

I am now 27 years old. I have found a "managing cocktail" that has been working well for me. I am still becoming familiar with this version of myself. Learning what "triggers" my RA flares. I'm familiar with my affected areas and the time it takes for my body to recover. I have adapted many "preventative methods." I am back to strutting in my heels at social events. I still have my days where my "managing cocktail" just isn't enough. I experience chronic fatigue and brain fog. I also have a prevalent secondary condition called hypothyroidism. Some days I limp. Some days I have to wrap my hand up.

Sometimes all I want is a heat pad. Sometimes I have to opt for compression socks with mules, or compression socks and crocs. In the near future I will continue pursuing my dreams and finally obtain my degree!

Fellow warriors, advocates and allies. I have shared a bit of my journey with you in the hopes that you see that although rheumatoid arthritis is NOT pretty, life can still be beautiful. I'm so thankful to God for everyone He allowed to help me and for "peace that surpasses all understanding."

I am embracing "new norms." RA and I aren't "besties" BUT we do have a balance going.

I guess you can call it "Poetic Disharmony."

These days you can find me blogging on Instagram by searching illest.chronicals. I have also started the hashtag, #RALooksLikeMeToo, which is a passion that has been ignited within me, to dismantle stereotypes and raise awareness about my "dynamic disability," and the vast variety of the "Spoonie Spectrum," because "RA is NOT one size fit all!"

Well wishes fellow warriors. May your flares be few and far between.

Mary Nathan

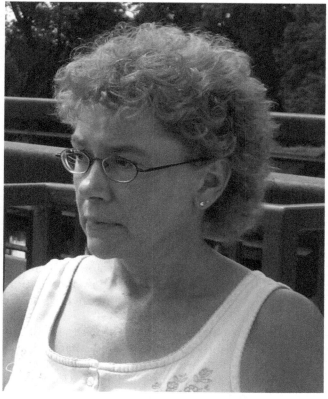

"Quieting My Soul."

Growing up as a pastor's daughter, I often felt like I had a red flashing arrow over my head. In grade school years, my older sister and I got into a shin-kicking, name-calling brawl, while walking home from school. A fuss budget parishioner, peering out her window, noticed. Mom knew of our antics by the time we got home. Apparently this was conduct unbecoming of the pastor's kids.

If being a pastor's daughter was like living in a fish bowl it was also where I learned about faith. My dad's faith was not of the fire and brimstone variety. He taught me of a loving, forgiving and gracious God. I saw my dad live his faith in the way he treated others. It wasn't just words on Sunday morning for him. It was a way of life, a way of interacting with the world. Although my dad died when I was 16, he sparked my interest in theology and spirituality.

During my college years, and early adulthood, I became what I refer to as a "lapsed Lutheran." Church attendance was not a regular part of my life but I sought the Divine through conversation with friends of all faiths, college courses, and books. God was very real to me both as a confidant and occasional target of my anger and angst.

For a few decades I was content to let my spiritual side hum quietly, the background music of my busy life of marriage, kids, work and caring for my mom.

At 42, I needed some minor shoulder surgery which evolved into needing a shoulder replacement at 44. I recovered and picked my life back up. But very soon my knees and hips were failing. They were all replaced in a span of three years. It seemed as if I was either in a lot of pain and needing surgery or recovering from surgery.

I watched a commercial for humira during that time and thought, *"Well, at least I don't need that."* I put that in the, "what a relief" category and tried to forget that my hands hurt, and that I was almost too tired some days to remember my name.

Throughout this time I was not testing positive for autoimmune arthritis. Then one morning a knuckle in my right hand looked like a golf ball. Several months and vials of blood later I was diagnosed with rheumatoid arthritis, which has since morphed into psoriatic arthritis.

Through the first few months after diagnosis I displayed every negative emotion possible, often several times a day. Drama and tears tended to increase as my doctor tried a variety of medications, most of which either didn't help, or caused unmanageable side effects. Ever been alone in the middle of a Walmart in white jeans with a full cart, a throbbing ankle, boiling intestines and an urgent need for a bathroom? I felt utter despair for what the rest of my life with autoimmune arthritis could potentially look like.

Family and friends remained supportive, but I knew that they weren't thrilled with the way I was handling myself. RA was the only thing on my mind and in every conversation. Some people began to distance themselves. I knew that if I didn't get a grip on the newly diagnosed me, RA had the potential to leave me a very lonely and bitter woman.

Part of me wanted to sit on the couch, Kleenex by my side, while I crippled up. I imagined myself as the hostess of a very long pity party. But some spark of hope stirred within me. It whispered,

"You can. You can rise to this challenge. Do it, if not for yourself, then do it for the people who love you." If my joints ached, and medications left me tired and nauseous, the me in me, my spirit, wanted something better.

Call it serendipitous, or a God wink, when a friend suggested we do a Bible study book together. The book's focus was how to manage changing emotions and circumstances by standing on God's promises and presence.

My casual daily practice of meditation and prayer began to stretch into a larger quest. Could this be a path to better emotional and mental health which would ripple into my physical health?

I was not seeking a miracle cure directly from Heaven, but something transformative. Could a deeper spirituality help me be well within my chronic illness? When the rug was pulled out from under me time and again at a doctor appointment, could I find a solid footing within my faith?

My adult approach to spirituality in general, and Christianity in particular, isn't conventional. I believe there are many ways to worship, many paths to the Divine.

I treasure many of the traditions of the Lutheran church; the liturgy of my childhood can bring tears to my eyes. I am also a seeker of new ways to express my faith.

I don't want to say hello to God on Sunday morning and forget about Him the rest of the week. If faith was to help me live with a chronic illness, I needed something more.

There are 17th century Pietists in my family tree. The Pietist movement emphasized a more personal relationship with God, a daily connection to the Divine. That appealed to me. I began to purposefully spend time each morning reading from a variety of devotions. I followed with some quiet moments. I let my mind search for God, while attempting to quiet my thoughts and the way they clamored at me to feel fear, worry, anger and grief over the way my life had changed.

My journal entries began to shape themselves into prayers, or at least conversations with God. Sometimes though, try as I might, I could not find a positive or thankful note to end on. But I was starting to grow some spiritual muscle and the peace that comes with it. People close to me noticed that things I would normally worry to a nubbin were not taking up space in my head.

Bigger storms were brewing though, externally and internally. The summer of 2019 hit me hard and threatened to derail the work I had done. My beloved brother died, a close friend had come close to death and my illness was not responding to the arsenal of drugs my rheumatologist threw at it. My disease remained severe and active.

Not content with attacking my joints, RA inflamed my eyes, a condition called uveitis. Daily steroid drops tamed that and then my hair began to fall out. I cried in the shower as clumps came out of the crusty lesions on my scalp. RA had evolved to PsA, a whole new beast to get to know.

I felt defeat and despair. I had no resources left to put lipstick on this particular pig, and I wasn't in the mood to make lemonade out of lemons.

God winked at me again in the form of a book about grace. The grace that I tried to extend to others was also my gift from God. God was willing to give me room to grieve and be angry. He'd stick around. God smiled at my joy on good days when I could inhabit my life without pain as a constant companion. God gave me courage to have another joint surgery and try yet another new medication. He didn't even mind that I complained about it. Often.

When I trusted God enough with all of my life, even the ugly parts, I found that He was always there. Here was my solid ground. I began to understand that God was not in my longing of what might have been, or in my fear of the future. He is in my here and now. He is in my day-to-day life with a painful chronic illness. And it's here, with knowledge of a loving and present Creator, that I can accept my illness and my changing physical limits. I also accept that I will not do this perfectly, but I strive to claim peace within a constantly changing medical journey.

The faith that teaches me to accept all of me, including my illness, has made me more available to others in a much more genuine way. I volunteer for the Arthritis Foundation. I want people to know that they are not alone. I want them to know that they are not crazy. This disease impacts all parts of our lives, physically, mentally and emotionally. There will be tough days but better days will come.

I keep note cards displayed at my desk with inspiring spiritual quotes. As I type this I read *"Quiet my soul that I might be where I am."* That's my motto now as I head off to another doctor's appointment, feel the sting of canceled plans, or just enjoy time with family and friends. My wish for you is that you too will find quiet for your soul!

Kristen Drennen

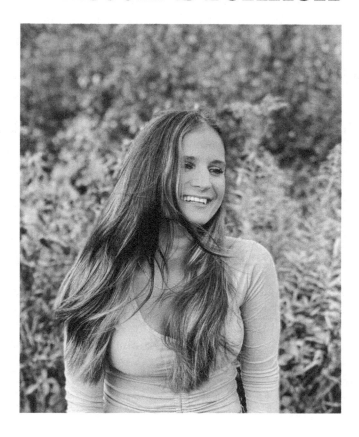

"Slow down and find joy in the little things. It really is some of the best medicine."

I've always loved cooking and preparing food for people ever since I was a little girl. It's been 11 years now since I've been diagnosed with rheumatoid arthritis (RA), which has made cooking a bit more of a challenge at times. Often I rely on my husband, or an electric jar opener to open bottles or jugs. Working with flour, as therapeutic as it is for me, is not always easy.

But I think that's the inspiration…doing that thing you're passionate about despite the setbacks or limitations.

My joints may still be deformed, but slowly I've experienced healing internally that surpasses any kind of physical healing. I used to place all of my worth and identity into my athleticism or how "healthy" I thought I was. When all of that was stripped away from years of eating disorders and RA, that's where I found freedom, and no longer place my worth and identity in those things. Usually we think of healing from arthritis as "physical," but I believe the healing I've experienced in my heart, and my mind, has given me more freedom and an even fuller life.

After trekking over seven miles of lava rock fields many years ago, I learned that when there isn't any worldly comfort within reach to take away the pain, it forces you to depend on God, who gives a spiritual comfort beyond anything this world can give. I remember lying there in the sand, on the furthest southern point in the United States, belly laughing so hard and feeling so secure, so loved, so taken care of.

This is where I find healing. This is where I find life, strength, and joy. Thankfulness even.

Do I believe in physical healing? Absolutely. And though sickness is not from God, do I also believe that he may use these struggles to refine us more into who we are meant to be? 1000%. I continue on giving thanks, because no matter how I feel or what my circumstances may be, He is still good, and He works all things together for the good.

Over the years I've become passionate about living a slower and simpler life. It truly helps me to manage the symptoms, and take care of myself, to live the best quality of life I can. I have two beautiful children (my little joys) who need a mother at her best. Not a perfect one, but a happy and healthy one.

I had exhausted myself rushing through my days that turned into years, trying to keep up with an eating disorder and manage RA. I was burnt out by my own doing, and now taking care of myself isn't even a question with two little ones in tow. Having an autoimmune disease, and raising a family, has brought me to this place of slowing down, and I'm grateful, cause this is where I found the fullest life. I see now how much life I missed out on in the rush.

This slower life put me in a position where I had to overcome a fear I've always had of letting others down. If I felt like I was, I could go on and on over-explaining myself. This people-pleasing mentality goes all the way back to when I first fell into an eating disorder at 12 years old. I am still very much learning to not let anxiety get the best of me in these moments of worrying what others are thinking, or wondering if what I can do is enough. The added stress or over-extending myself is certainly not worth the cost of a flare. When I feel like I'm being pulled in all different directions, and the fear creeps in of letting people down if I can't attend or do this or that, all I have to do is look at my kids' faces. I'm reminded why I have healthy limits and say no when my body is saying no.

My children made me realize how much of a gift our time truly is...a priceless and irreplaceable gift. It's up to me if I'm going to squander it or take the counter-cultural way of "busyness and haste" and instead, pursue to steward this one life well, and to the fullest...with or without RA.

Living with a chronic condition can certainly bring you to this place of stewarding your time more wisely. To savor the moments instead of rushing them away. To prioritize what you value most. To give and do what you can with joy, and know that it is enough. To teach my kids to live their lives intentionally. To not miss all the little blessings that God has woven into the mundane and routine.

My hope for anyone reading this is that you would be inspired to slow down and find joy in the little things. It really is some of the best medicine. And lastly, be encouraged that maybe you are healing in a much bigger way than you could have ever imagined.

Christina Moore

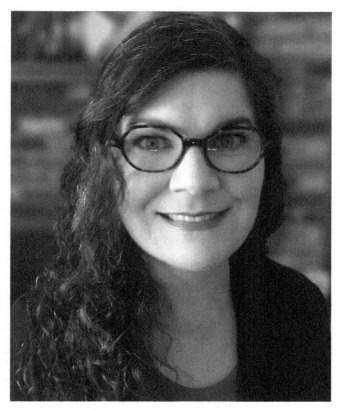

"Chronic illnesses take much from us, but they give unexpected gifts to us too."

The Thai rheumatologist looked at my husband. *"Culture shock,"* he said. *"There's nothing wrong with her but culture shock. Just push her through the first year or two and she'll be fine."* At my husband's side, I was too stunned for words. Could that really explain all the strange things happening in my body? Was it all in my head?

Three years prior to that conversation, I met my beloved at a missions prayer meeting at our church. We discovered we were both students at the same theological school preparing for missions. At school we became friends, then more than friends, bound by love of the Lord, good books, worship music, and teaching the Bible cross-culturally. When he proposed to me, we knew he was heading to the mission field soon, possibly within six months; we decided to marry before that so we could learn the culture and language together. Everything about our courtship, engagement, and newlywed life served that goal. We purged our belongings and only registered for the bare essentials needed to function in our apartment until we moved to Southeast Asia. In reality, our preparations took a year and a half, during which we traveled frequently, building our support teams, training church leaders at home and abroad, and visiting family we would not see for several years. We also spent dozens of hours at coffee shops, mentoring younger friends, writing for our ministry newsletter, planning Bible studies, or relaxing together. We took in as much beautiful green space and live music as we could, stockpiling memories for life on the other side of the world.

One unexpected challenge was obtaining health insurance with international coverage. During our engagement I had lost 25 pounds (10 more than my doctor preferred). A prior endometriosis diagnosis had required one surgery but was well-controlled, and my blood pressure was chronically low. My diet was as healthy as we could afford, and I ran or walked several miles six days a week. That preexisting chronic illness brought refusals from company after company until the very last option. They accepted us, and we accelerated our preparations for our move to Bangkok for the first four or five years of the rest of our lives overseas. Meanwhile, my fingers had started turning blue when I was cold. I knew that was called Raynaud's phenomenon, but nothing else seemed wrong, so we plowed on towards our calling and dream.

In 2001, we moved to downtown Bangkok. We learned public transportation and navigated unfamiliar streets and menus. We enrolled in language school and joined a church. Culture shock brought many tears, quests for familiar foods and quiet garden spaces, long sessions alone with God and my books, and computer-gaming sessions for my husband. That was normal. What was not normal was that my fingers continued to turn blue, my hands often hurt, I ran a low fever for hours daily, my pulse raced and I couldn't climb the stairs to the Sky Train without help. Then the vertigo began. Without warning, the room would suddenly spin like a top set in motion. That was the first symptom that really scared me.

We found an internist who spoke fluent English. She drew vials and vials of blood and determined liver and inflammation markers were very elevated. Combined with my symptoms, *"It might be lupus,"* she said. *"You need to see a rheumatologist."* The rheumatologist ran more tests and diagnosed culture shock. Not satisfied, we kept returning for more tests, asking physicians stateside what to request. Hundreds of people around the world, from the church secretary to a visiting Anglican bishop, were praying for my healing. To all appearances, things were getting worse, not better.

"Fibromyalgia," the rheumatologist said with a wave of his hand. "Nothing you can do." Research showed us the definitive symptom was specific tender points throughout the body. Which I didn't have. We consulted a neurologist. He ruled out brain-based causes of the vertigo and echoed the first doctor, *"All your symptoms look like lupus. Your labs don't fit the textbook profile, but if it quacks like a duck..."* By that time we had already reached the same conclusion and were taking steps toward returning to the United States. If it was lupus, it would be lifelong, and we would need our community for the journey. Also, Bangkok was replete with the environmental lupus triggers.

My husband faced the choice of sacrificial faithfulness to our marriage covenant, to love and serve me like Jesus, or his vocational dream from long before we met. In perhaps the noblest decision of his life, he chose me. He laid down his felt calling to keep his marriage vows.

That kind neurologist provided basic care until we moved back to Texas. At our first specialist appointment after returning, the day before my birthday, the new rheumatologist told me I did indeed have systemic lupus erythematosus (SLE). We began treatment with several prescription medicines, and my physical health slowly stabilized.

Emotionally, however, we were broken, ashamed, and disoriented. We were the regional team leaders for our mission organization, with several other aspiring missionaries preparing to join us overseas. Our hard choice affected their futures too. The missions program we worked for had no employment opportunities for my husband in the home office, but God provided through a previous employer who created a technology position especially for him. We were grateful for that gift and also struggling to get our feet under us after this huge plot twist. We faced overwhelming grief, but family and the quiet worship of our new church home helped us through.

One characteristic of autoimmune diseases, unhappily, is the flare and remission cycle. After approximately seven years of medication-induced remission, a surgery destabilized my lupus. Out of the blue, intense chest pain leveled me. Any pressure on my sternum at all was agonizing. Breathing hurt unless I lay down on my side. For many sofa-bound months, fatigue was so debilitating that I texted my mom before and after I showered so someone would know if I passed out washing my hair.

By the time my rheumatologist found a medication that helped the chest pain, other joints chimed in, one after another, like petulant children demanding attention. At our wits' end, we sought a second opinion, and "undifferentiated inflammatory arthritis" was added to my chronic illness portfolio. The new doctor felt that joint pain had become too prominent a symptom to be attributable to lupus alone. A few more specific arthritis labels have been considered since, but that big umbrella diagnosis is enough to access care.

Chronic illness has taken so much from me: health, hobbies, exercise, friendships, a church community, family time, special occasions, independence. My invisible illness has often left me feeling invisible. Most painful of all was the loss of my husband's and my shared vocation, the only thing we wanted to do, the thing we believed God called us to do.

But that's not the whole story. Chronic illness has also given much.

Chronic illness is teaching me courage, by leading me straight into my biggest fears, and showing me I can survive them because God is with me.

Chronic illness is teaching me perseverance, by placing me in a difficult situation where all the emergency exits are locked. In accepting this and looking for good even here, I am learning to find peace and trust God's goodness.

Chronic illness is teaching me gratitude, by putting entitlement to death. No one appreciates simple pleasures like the person who endures extended periods when they are out of reach.

Chronic illness is teaching me the humility of saying on a daily basis, *"I can't do this. Will you help me?"* In a do-more, climb-higher, run-faster world, arthritis and lupus slow me down and force me to discern what is really mine from the Lord to do.

Chronic illness has tenderized my heart toward the pain of others. It is easier to weep with those who weep and rejoice with those who rejoice, and broken hearts seem to find safe harbor with me. My shattering has made room for the shattered stories of others, and there are so very many shattered souls who need shelter.

Finally, chronic illness has given me new friends and purpose through the blog my husband helped me start during those laid-flat sofa months. Chronic illness took me from one mission field and opened a new one.

If you, dear reader, are facing a new arthritis diagnosis, or waiting anxiously for one, grieve your losses when they come. They matter. Grief honors that. Chronic illnesses take much from us, but they give unexpected gifts to us too. May you face your plot twist with eyes wide open to both and have courage to face them. Life will never be the same, but it can be good and beautiful again.

Mary Ann Matteson Buchan

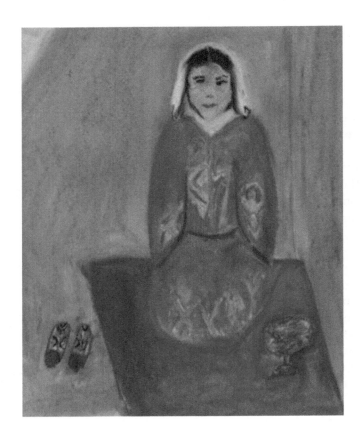

"Never give up, never give in."

The importance of daily prayers and meditation, in helping alleviate a chronic illness such as rheumatoid arthritis, cannot be underestimated. Many sufferers have anxiety, stressors and hopelessness. It is a most difficult disorder for physicians to diagnose and treat with efficacy. My personal experience was one plagued with questions , symptoms that could be explained away as aches and pains . I first went in for treatment in 2004, my hands swollen, my joints aching, yet it was not taken seriously. Blood tests were taken, and despite my vigorous protests, nothing was done. I told anyone who would listen that my family had a history of arthritis, and the cacophony of *"yeah so,"* from physicians, nurses and practitioners, made it a very harrowing ordeal. *"Take an Aleve, you will feel better. Lose some weight and exercise. We all have pain."* Not like this.

For those of you unfamiliar with the intricacies of RA, it is nothing like arthritis we may experience as we age. Some people have osteoarthritis. I have both. That being said, I kept searching for answers. While always nutritionally aware I had gained quite a lot of weight. I knew the pressure on my joints wasn't good so I lost over 150 pounds through diet and exercise. I thought I had pulled a muscle doing some stretches one morning on my daily walk. *"Top of the morning,"* I'd say to the passers by. I would go to work and stand for 8-10 hours and go home in pain. This went on for years.

I finally asked a doctor to run every blood panel they could at the clinic. I had no health insurance at the time. In 2015 I was diagnosed with RA. I was relieved that I had a diagnosis. Having come from a background in medicine, my grandfather was a chief surgeon, I sought out ways to treat the symptoms. I applied for disability. My doctor stated *"here's methotrexate, take this you will feel much better."* I took one dose and my tongue was swollen, anaphylactic shock. Oh no.

This began my journey into treatment, finding the right physicians and years of trial and error. The side effects of medication can cause other problems. Standardized treatments did not work well for me. I fine tuned my diet . The medication caused mouth sores. I have ulnar drift and need a knee replacement. I have a slight moon face from prednisone and gained some weight (not much). *"How's your Cortisol burnout?"* *"Hey cripple."* These are a reflection of their souls, their lack of kindness and compassion. God gave me kindness. I am a nurturing loving woman with a sense of wonder and a great sense of humor. I made indelible friendships! All throughout this excruciating pain, and when I say excruciating I mean excruciating, I prayed. It is the gift of a lifetime.

My mom gave me her rosary collection from our family. I am a Catholic. It is how I have gotten through this. My belief in God is so strong that nothing can come between my faith and my optimistic attitude. When faced with flares I pray. I don't get brain fog, nor am I depressed. When that burden is shared it is the courage and wisdom moving me forward. I know for a fact that God will hear me. I have had the very worst of medical care, and I did not acquiesce. I refused pain medication where I almost died from anemia. Finding that balance takes courage, these are cancer drugs, not for sissies.

Soul strength. My greatest form of treatment comes from greeting every day in prayer and giving thanks to God. Miracles do happen. I have handled each situation with God given grace. I know peace. I am a very happy person because of God's love. He puts just the right people in your life. I have that wisdom. Don't be afraid to ask for God's help and blessings. All great things begin and end with the Lord. He is the alpha and omega.

And it does not hurt to double up on omega 3's. Vitamins are necessary in replacing lost nutrients and believe me when I say grow your own veggies, or buy organic, because as a friend says *"we are under toxic environmental attack and we must heal our gut and our microbiome."* I hope in my lifetime we find the cure for autoimmune disorders. They are on the rise. Until then I turn to the greatest healer I know, Jesus Christ. He sustains my soul. A fountain of strength in turbulence. My father was a decorated war hero and as I always say God is my copilot. Never give up, never give in. God has a beautiful plan for us in the land of the living.

Thank you and may God bless and keep you in his stead.

Elii Chapman

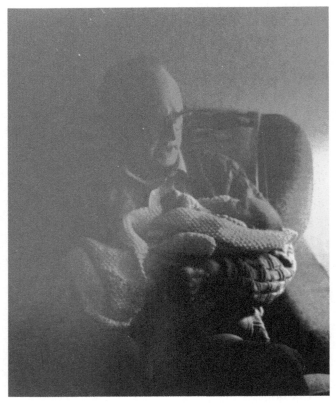

"It (rheumatoid arthritis) may change over time, but for now, use of the various tools I have in my toolbox brings me a feeling of empowerment."

Every Other Generation

In the photo my paternal grandpa is holding my baby daughter in 1992. The deformity of one of his hands is minimally visible in the low light. This is the only picture that I have of him that includes his hands. Rheumatoid arthritis destroyed the joints of his fingers and toes, but it also resulted in the utter devastation of his tendons and ligaments.

While growing up, I watched the impact of this disease on the lives of my grandparents, but the thought of touching my life never crossed my mind.

The beginning of 2021 meant the beginning of my fourth quarter of unanticipated online teaching. I woke on the first day of the new year with what I thought was a developing bunion on my left foot. By the middle of January I was walking every morning, to my living room work station, to Zoom with the students for the morning. Each day, the pain in the ball of one foot was mirrored more intensely in the other. Teaching on February mornings became more challenging as the pain began to emerge in my hands, again first the left, then the right. This was obviously not an injury. Teaching online granted me flexibility of time. Research began after the last Zoom each day. By the middle of February, I called my primary care doctor and asked her to make an exception and order tests for many things prior to seeing me, in addition to the rheumatoid factor, to give us a thorough set of data to discuss at our online appointment. She was willing. A few weeks later, after we discussed my low positive rheumatoid factor, I had my referral to a rheumatologist and would see him the week before returning to in-person teaching. The week of my Spring Break included getting the classroom ready, giving myself my first subcutaneous dose of methotrexate, and my 50th birthday. It was clear that due to the pandemic, this was a historic year, but for me, it meant I had work to do. It was time to find all the tools in my context that I could use to make this work within my definition of life.

Advice from my sister in law on manual self-injection... *"Just do it like you are ripping off a band-aid."* That worked. Elimination diet efforts, when I had already been an organic vegetarian nearly half my life...reduce intake of bread, really try to avoid sugar but otherwise keep the routine. More research had to be done on that >500+ anti-CCP result. A couple years of chronic sinus infections ended that summer with surgery on my deviated septum.

MOVE, move, move. My first morning with pain free feet was followed by an afternoon where I delivered a thank you card, and awesome socks, to my primary care nurse practitioner, who used to be a school nurse (I've got to add). My visit with a podiatrist added to the list:

achilles tendonitis, heel bone spurs, plantar fasciitis, and eight degree pronate angles in both ankles. By November, without changing my nutritional intake much, nor my physical output much, I had lost thirty pounds and had blood work ordered to check for diabetes or thyroid issues. The conclusion: that was 30 pounds of swelling. The year of 2021 came to a finale on the rough side, with three insurance denials for a prescription move to a biologic, and lastly a call from the dermatologist, to set an appointment for basal cell carcinoma removal. Well, if given the choice of types of cancer, that's the one I'd choose for sure! Happy New Year!

Not far into the second semester we had a partial class quarantine. That morning I found out that a section of the class needed to be invited to Zoom for math. Technical trouble dominated the day. The kids on Zoom couldn't hear me. While the students in class waited so patiently, I checked all the cables, then the settings, then closed and re-started Zoom, but didn't succeed until rebooting the computer. During all this I could feel my knee begin to swell. The lucky thing that day was a scheduled follow-up appointment at the rheumatologist office with perfect timing. Between 11:00 a.m. and 3:30 p.m. my knee became the size of a cantaloupe. It was treated right then and there and the next day was another sick day.

Motivation to find the right medication is what gets one through the months of medication that is ineffective, and the months of medication that adds to the pain. Trying to sleep in a body that is so uncomfortable to live in requires so much energy, that's not how sleep works. One medication brought two new issues, the experience of the urge to itch, so great that scratching could feel euphoric, and also UV sensitivity so severe that sunlight exposure was equivalent to having acid poured on the skin. All this just meant seeing a dermatologist for more tools.

This past school year, my 14th year, resulted in more sick days than my cumulative career. The tools I have used include Mediterranean recipes, Hoka shoes with custom orthotic inserts, various supplements, physical therapy, cortisone injections under the kneecap and in both ankles, compression gloves and foot sleeves, and CBD topical gel. Prescribed medications have included prednisone, methotrexate, sulfasalazine, leflunomide, and humira. The last two weeks of the school year, sulfasalazine was leaving my system. The side effect resulted in cracks in the skin of most of the joints in my fingers. I had to wear band aids to prevent getting blood on student work.

Last month, my hope returned. After school let out, my husband and I went to three Hawaiian islands for two weeks. I brought swim wear that covered everything from the neck down. I bought two bottles of sunscreen from the dermatologist's office. I was continuing with leflunomide as the side effects wore off, and brought the prednisone for when the symptoms returned. According to my smart watch, I walked an average of 60+ miles each of those two weeks. I snorkeled four times and saw so much wildlife. I slept well and felt treasured. When I got home, I had a week to get ready for the summer camp I had signed up to host at the school where I teach. This was also something else that had never crossed my mind. I was going to be paid $35 an hour to roller skate.

As the funding was coming from the state, I needed to have some academic standards to assess at the beginning and end of the camp. I grew up roller skating, but I had never learned about the Newtonian physics of it. A summer skate camp was exactly what I needed after being masked in a classroom for a school year. We learned the physics of movement together with comprehension that came from the kinesthetic experience. The assessment score average at the beginning of camp was 24% and average at the end of camp was 80%.

The challenge of this disease is something new and different every day. It is utterly unpredictable, but there are many things that can be done to try to gain control over the effects. It may change over time, but for now, use of the various tools I have in my toolbox, brings me a feeling of empowerment.

Elisabeth Abeson

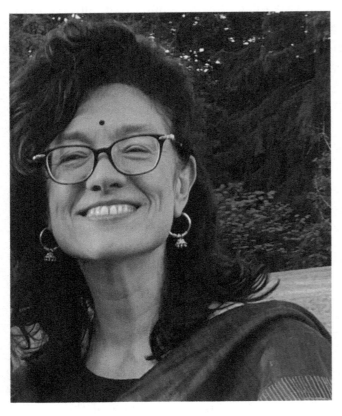

"My Altar Buddies."

I don't mean any disrespect by calling the Gods, Goddess, and the venerable Monk on my altar, 'my buddies'. Sure, I bow, pray and light incense for them, but those aren't the most sacred moments. The most sacred ones are those in which I let down my self-sufficiency guard and allow these enlightened souls to metaphorically hold my hand - supporting me in partnership. Albeit, it is kind of an unequal partnership as I am a mere earthling, but I feel taken care of none-the-less. Just like 'the buddy system' at camp, we're in it together. They have my back and I'm grateful.

It's no wonder I ventured out into the spiritual realm. RA wreaked havoc on my body and the co-morbidity of depression wore heavily on my mind. As things weren't too comfortable in these earth-bound areas of my 'hood, I needed to hijack it out of there to make sense of what was going on...and to find respite.

The year I was diagnosed with RA was the year I deepened my spirituality. It is not like I had 'get spiritual' on my to-do list and sat in a different temple, church, mosque or forest weekly until I felt the vibe. No, nothing like that. Instead, what was on my to-do list was to find a healing modality for treating my sero-positive RA holistically - on the level of body, mind and spirit. It felt instinctively right for me, and was reinforced by the fact that my mom went down the allopathic path, for her RA, and it didn't end well.

So, I ventured out into trying different approaches that were available to me in the States. Homeopathic medicine, naturopathic medicine and traditional chinese medicine, were the lowest hanging fruits that seemed ripe for the pickin'. I read scores of papers and books, consulting with doctors whose work was based on the most discerning evidence-based research. In keeping with my overachieving ways, I was a judiciously compliant patient. Nothing got me feeling well enough to walk easefully, so I literally limped along until I came across a double-blind, randomized, controlled, pilot study that compared methotrexate with classic ayurvedic medicine for RA.

The people who were treated with ayurvedic medicine did as well with far fewer side effects, so my interest was piqued. I ended up becoming a patient of the principal investigators (PI) for both the allopathic and ayurvedic teams. Six months later, I arrived at the PI's Ayurvedic Hospital, in southern India, and was surprised to find it was built around a temple dedicated to the Lord of Healing.

Like any seasoned patient with a systemic chronic illness, I see lots of doctors. Lots of specialists. So, I am used to wings of hospitals being dedicated to exceedingly wealthy families, and to courtyards at integrative health centers, having an Americanized "Zen" theme with a water wall abutting some well-manicured bamboo. But, actually building a hospital around a bonafide temple, staffed with real, live religious figures, was way outside what I had ever experienced. It was like a new frontier.

I felt like a starship enterprise crew member, encountering something worthy of a season finale. Some mind-blowingly new world - something so different that I didn't have the vocabulary to describe it. I stared, I watched, I smelled the scents coming from the temple, and I heard sounds that seemed strikingly important to those that sung them. I was jet-lagged and a tad overwhelmed, but I was strangely drawn to, and comforted by, the extravaganza.

Fast forward 10 years. I have courted the extravaganza metaphorically for a decade. The early years showcased evidence-based healing on the level of the Body. I could walk easefully again, had far fewer flares, and eventually attained remission. Additionally, my dry eyes from Sjogren's syndrome were no longer keeping me up at night and I felt like I had a new lease on life. It was as if someone lowered the heat significantly on my body's thermostat. No longer was my furnace operating at crisis level.

Then, there was healing on the level of the mind. I came to terms with childhood abuse that seemed to release its grip on my tissues, muscles and bones as my system detoxified at the cellular level through the ayurvedic healing process. Indeed, as Bessel Van der Kolk reminds us so eloquently, "The Body Keeps the Score." Yup, indeed, my 'vessel' knew exactly what it had been through, and my reprieve on the level of physical pain freed up enough energetic resources for me to acknowledge, grieve and honor the degree to which my body had been impacted by emotional suffering.

And, then there was healing on the level of the Spirit - an ethereal realm that I escaped to throughout life when my body and mind were under siege. It was a place where I made art, spun stories and connected to something bigger than the sum of my parts. This place made me feel connected to water, to nature, to animals, to beings so benevolent that some called them Gods. I consider myself spiritual and view religion as multi-denominational - all leading to the same tenets that the global community strives to live by and, sometimes, attain.

Personally, I am drawn to Engaged Buddhism in the practice of Thich Nhat Hanh, and the Buddha has presided over my home altar along with Thay's soothing smile for decades. But the year I was diagnosed with RA, and treated with Ayurvedic medicine so successfully, Thay gained altar buddies. The first was the Lord of Healing, Dhanvantari - the God orchestrating the earlier-mentioned extravaganza in the Ayurvedic hospital's temple.

Initially, I did not identify with Lord Dhanvantari given his multiple arms holding things as varied as a leech, a conch shell and some herbs. But he was the deity that presided over the treatment room where I went from limping to walking, to healing emotionally, and to reuniting with art and writing in the realm of spirit. Given all this, Lord Dhanvantari's presence really grew on me.

I was struck by the fact that the Massage Team leader cupped medicinal oil in her hands, and chanted to this God before applying it on my head. They also lit a candle at the feet of his framed image on the wall and did something in concert with the internal medicines, daily regimens and diet to make my pain go away. Not just pain within the jurisdiction of one specialist, but whole-body pain.

So, what was going on here? My mom's infusion room nurse never prayed before administering her biologic. And, my mom was never pain-free. Was there a link? I soon started humming what the massage team chanted, as I associated the sounds with the outpouring of care they gave me. It was self-soothing. I didn't understand what they were saying, but I did feel the energy the sounds imparted and knew it contributed significantly to my healing.

So, I got a little picture of Lord Dhanvantari on my wall and lit my own candle to him in the evenings. I prayed for good health and thanked him for watching over me. It felt good to relinquish some of my strong-willed control over to someone else. I had faith in my doctor, the medicine, the massage team, the nurses the chemists and now...a multi-armed man that seemed to be at the top of this hierarchical healing community. It made me feel a part of something larger. I was not Hindu, but as Lord Dhanvantari derives from this rich tradition, I was an enthusiastically respectful devotee. His healing methods were pioneeringly elegant and focused on addressing the root cause of suffering, rather than masking it. I liked this healing modality, so it was time for Thay and the Buddha to be joined by another venerable altar buddy.

Such an impressive coterie of beings graced my altar now - Thay, Buddha, Lord Dhanvantari, and a Goddess named Saraswati. As the Hindu Goddess of art, culture, music, learning and literature, she was my kind of gal. A fine arts major in undergrad, I identified as an artist, but took a 25-year sabbatical. It was not until I had healed enough on the level of body and mind, that I had the inner resources to venture into the spiritual realm and reunite with art.

I did this through expressive arts therapy when I was a patient, by creating a mixed media collage from Ayurvedic materials I found in the hospital and its healing temple. It was the perfect way for me to transform treatment discomfort into something positive. From then on, Saraswati had renewed importance in my life. I was drawn to her presence to bring out the artful soul in me...just as I was drawn to Lord Dhanvantari to remind me of my body's own capacity to heal. Holding hands with my altar buddies on either side, I truly knew how to find my way home.

Dañiela Grisel

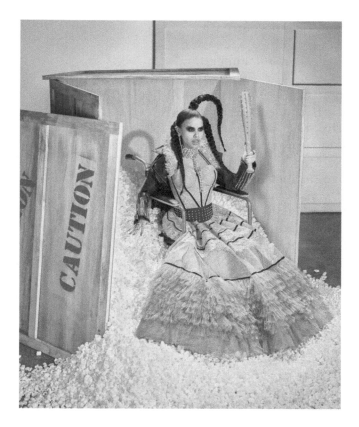

"If you ever feel alone because of your pain from rheumatoid arthritis, remember that you're not alone, you were never alone and you'll never be alone, because there is an entire community that understands your pain."

If you have rheumatoid arthritis I understand your pain. If you feel the burning, stabbing, throbbing, piercing pain throughout every inch of your body, then I understand your pain. If you have to live your life in this chronic pain 24/7, I understand your pain.

If the joints in your hands hurt from reading this book, I understand your pain. If you get a flare up, every time you eat your favorite snacks, then I understand your pain. If you get told by doctors that you're lying about being in chronic pain, while being in chronic pain, I understand your pain. If you get told that you're "faking it" by family, friends and strangers, then I understand your pain.

If your prescription for RA causes side effects but you need it to manage your pain, then I understand your pain. If your pain is always being dismissed because "you're always in pain", then I understand your pain. If people make you feel like a burden because you need help doing simple tasks because your joints are completely inflamed and you're in chronic pain, then I understand your pain.

If you always have to cancel plans with

friends because you're in too much pain, then I understand your pain. If you've asked yourself and God, "WHY ME!?", then I understand your pain. If you've cried yourself to sleep too many times to count, then I understand your pain.

If you can't hold your own child because of how much your body hurts, then I understand your pain.

If you can no longer walk because your body turned against itself, then I understand your pain. If your entire life has completely changed because of rheumatoid arthritis, then I understand your pain.

If you ever feel alone because of your pain from rheumatoid arthritis, remember that you're not alone, you were never alone and there is an entire community that understands your pain.

If you have rheumatoid arthritis, I understand your pain.

PHYSICAL

Stories

Lauren Brooke

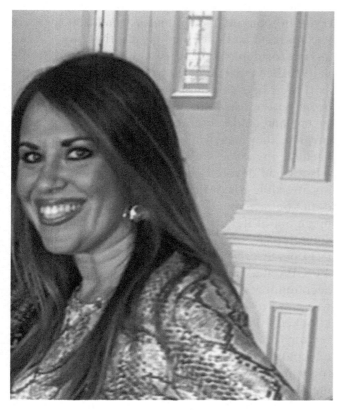

"The true agonizing journey of a sixteen year search for a diagnosis."

**Undiagnosed: My Sixteen Year Search
To Find My Arthritis Diagnosis**

Solutions to questions and problems provide equilibrium. They give a sense of certainty and acceptance. By not having this, it is potentially the worst part of finding yourself in a medical mystery. How so? It's exactly what defines the word mystery. The unknown. The worry behind the symptoms. The constant questioning of what is it? The talks you have with yourself in your mind as you try to decipher clues to find a solution. The dread of coming up empty and continuing on with pain that has no end in sight. A wish that you could just find an answer to your problem and that it could be simply fixed with a quick remedy.

Yet, no matter how hard you try — you can't. Your control is gone. This is what happened to me at age 15 to 31. Sixteen years of pain, disappointment, frustration, loneliness, and the yearn for an explanation.

You may ask, how does a 15-year-old girl handle this? I navigated my situation through the use of soul-crushing perseverance. I thought long and hard about the cliche saying, everything happens for a reason. When I think of my own journey, I quickly say it doesn't apply to me. But the question remains — does it?

It is daunting to think the latter could be true, but in some fashion it is. Perhaps, it was to share this very story with an audience who would no longer feel alone. Who would not feel that their pain is originating in their mind and who could finally put to rest the voices of others, who tried to silence or invalidate them. Maybe it's to tell a reader to never give up. My hope is to highlight the importance of adversity in the darkest of hours, days, and even years. When it could seem easy or the right thing to do; to surrender to a mystery — it is not. One must continue to find the light at the end of the tunnel and that is exactly what I did.

At age fifteen my life changed permanently. I remember the day my heel pain arrived so clearly. It was a crisp fall day and the sun was shining. Except, I did not know that the sun would begin to fade for me and my world would be muddled with darkness for the next decade and a half. I started to get dressed for school that morning when I began to feel intense pain in both of my feet. As the day continued and the pain lasted all throughout my school day, I knew something was wrong. This symptom marked the beginning of what would be a very dark period of my life.

The following weeks and months ahead were filled with sheer confusion and the beginning of trying to define my mysterious pain. From doctors and specialists, who misdiagnosed me with various conditions, to painful foot injections; my life as I had known it had disappeared. All of my diagnostic tests came with negative results, but I could no longer stand or walk without severe heel pain and agonizing burning sensations. I looked fine on the outside, but was drowning under the waves of pain that replicated like painful hot currents in my feet. I did not limp, but I had to find a seat within a few minutes of weight bearing. I had about five minutes until the pain would begin. Only five minutes!

I recall one particularly disturbing doctor visit to an orthopedic specialist, who told me that he had no idea what was causing my pain and that I would probably have to live with it forever. He explained that for the amount my insurance paid him, he had spent enough time on my case. I still cannot fathom how you tell a 16-year-old girl that she could never walk again without pain, discriminate against her insurance as a way of validating your resistance to help, and be able to look at yourself in the mirror. It was then that I began to learn how cruel and callous people can be, including doctors whom we place our trust in.

Additionally, I found myself alone and isolated. My weekends were no longer filled with outings—the invitations had ceased. The pain had stolen my friendships. Teenagers have difficulty understanding ongoing pain that doesn't have an expiration date. At school, I could no longer walk the stairs and had to take the elevator instead. I couldn't walk to the bus, so a van for handicapped students would drive me home. Everything had changed. I wasn't a healthy teen anymore. I was sick and misunderstood.

Each doctor I visited told me the importance of finding a comfortable shoe to wear to ease my pain. Yet, nothing was comfortable. When I say nothing, I truly mean it—shoes were now my arch nemesis. It's crazy to think that shoes can hold so much power in one's life, but they did. My feet had become so sensitized from the pain that every single shoe, no matter how comfortable it was supposed to be, was beyond uncomfortable. My mother and I would go to stores and spend hours trying on various types of footwear.

I remember the stacks of shoes that the salesperson would bring out in the hopes I would say yes to at least one pair, but I couldn't. Literally every pair increased my heel pain and burning. But more than the salesperson's disappointment, was mine and my mother's. We would go in with such high hopes that we would find the shoe that would ease my pain and I could be me again. I think we believed we would magically find this pair of shoes that I would put on my feet and I would be able to walk and stand again. Yet, we never could, no matter our efforts.

Unfortunately, the vicious cycles of empty doctor appointments went on for years. Treatments, therapies, shoes, inserts, medications did not alleviate the intense heel pain. I spent so much time trying to convince each doctor I met that the pain was real and had to defend myself that this was not anxiety or depression. It is sad that many chronic pain patients, particularly women, are often treated as if their pain is stemming from their mind. I had been put on several antidepressant medications to try and make me accept the pain. It was no surprise they never helped improve my condition, because the issue was physical and never mental. Also, I had devoted countless energy to defending my invisible disability to friends and family who didn't believe me. People thought I was making too much out of it, but looking back I never even made enough of it.

I persevered through college and maintained a 4.0 GPA at a prestigious university. I had handicap accommodations, parking spots, and my dorm room was close to the cafeteria and bathroom. Although I looked like a typical college student, my body felt anything but the sort. I eventually found a pair of sandals that were somewhat tolerable for me to wear. I would wear these sandals every day, no matter the climate. When it became cold, I would wear them with socks. Rain and snow; sandals were on. I recall going into the bathroom before my college classes to air dry my wet socks and would sometimes experience frost bitten toes from the cold. Yet, I could not change shoes due to my foot sensitivity. Academically college was great, but physically it was a very difficult and stressful time for me.

Upon college graduation, the search to find a solution became my sole focus. I could no longer try and pretend to live a normal life, because it wasn't. The pain became even more debilitating. If I went shopping, I would use a wheelchair to help me. The pain was ruining any kind of successful future. As my journey went on, and the doctor visits increased, it looked as if I would never find the reason for my symptoms. Except, at age 31 I did and everything changed.

Despite seeing many specialists, including rheumatologists, who told me I did not have inflammatory arthritis; I did. In fact, a form of autoimmune inflammatory arthritis was the cause of my severe heel pain. Specifically, it was diagnosed as spondyloarthritis, also known as SpA. I finally had a way to treat my pain. My journey was far from over, but my quest for an answer had ended.

Even though I had to accept that I had a chronic disease, I felt relieved. The pain that I had suffered was validated and recognized. It was real and even had a name. Instead of feeling like the only person in the world with these symptoms, it was an identifiable disease that others had. The answer to my entrapment had arrived which allowed me to be free.

Berina Kapa

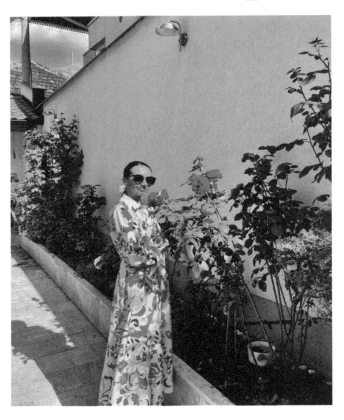

"Put yourself and your health first and you will keep rheumatoid arthritis under control. A lesson from my own experience!"

I live in Bosnia and Herzegovina. I am 45 years old and have been fighting rheumatoid arthritis for nine years.

I could be a medical example of how an RA patient could reach the disability phase in only 10 years from diagnosis, if you don't work continuously and adequately on your own health and wellbeing. After so many years, I am now dependent on my family members for basic life activities like getting dressed, cooking and cleaning.

My physical condition today is that I have visible deformities in my hands (ulnar deviation), wrists, elbows, shoulders and feet. At the beginning, only hands and fingers were deformed but other joints were damaged over years, especially during the pandemic phase when I spent most time at home.

So, let me tell you what you should do if recently diagnosed, to not come into the phase I am currently in. You can live with RA pretty normally with healthy anti-inflammatory food, regular moving and exercises and adequate medications.

Well, let's start with medications. Every patient reacts on medications differently and explores which is the best one for her/himself. In my case, proper medication therapy came a little late due to other diagnoses, like anemia and liver issues. I couldn't start with a higher methotrexate dose because I was underweight (due to a lot of pain) and couldn't cope with nausea, which was the main side-effect of this medication. So my hands were deformed and I got ulnar deviation pretty fast, within two years. Later on, I continued with a lower dose of methotrexate, even tried one biologic, but it didn't work in my case. Despite hand deformities, in the second year, I was pretty close to remission, thanks to herbal remedies I used so far (various detox teas and tinctures). This is just to remind you that alternative ways also work if you have a herbal specialist who can help you, depending on your overall condition and medications you take. In the third year, I started with one biologic medication which worked well for a couple of months, but later on didn't give results in my case, so I continued with methotrexate. I was afraid that there was no proper therapy for me back then, but obviously I should try some other. It is simply the matter of finding the right one for you together with your doctor. I will probably go with the new one.

Anyway, as you can conclude, prompt and adequate therapy is essential for getting RA patients on the right path and keeping her/him functioning normally. Find a good rheumatologist and speak about the best medication therapy for you. Explore it, keep in contact with your doctor and even write how you feel. Today, there are so many medications, especially biologics which help RA patients to function pretty well and live like there is no RA.

Let me tell you more about food and exercises. Please don't let yourself come into a situation like myself to ask yourself a question: Why didn't I do this before? Yes, I am asking myself this question because, for so many years, I made excuses that I cannot go on a diet or do exercises because I would experience a lot of joint pain, or I'd say I would do it tomorrow after I rest. You simply NEED to put yourself first place. Nothing else is important except your own health, nothing. I was working so hard, building my career despite everything, just to escape from my health problem, instead of focusing on how to improve it.

Eating anti-inflammatory food doesn't mean you need to go on a diet. It means you need to explore by yourself what food is good for your inflammation and pain, and which is not. Nobody can tell you that until you explore it on your own. And yes, you can see results. Unfortunately I realized that pretty late. Also, include more vegetables, fruits, nuts, seeds, fish and water in your nutrition. It doesn't need to be expensive either. If you can afford it, try to connect with a certified dietitian who can help you. You will be surprised if I tell you that recently I opened an instagram account where I post my healthy meals, mostly breakfasts, because I can do that at least without family help. I found a hobby and finally ate healthy.

And now we come to exercise. I know, you need motivation like myself. I never exercised regularly during these nine years. Yes, I walked and was active, but I was not having regular exercise. That also caused muscle atrophy and even worse joint pain and damage, because I didn't move often and strengthen my muscles, especially in the pandemic period. So I paid a price and am now trying to get back overall body strength. Maybe you will ask how to do fitness, pilates or yoga when in pain. Well, you would be surprised how many RA patients today are certified trainers because it helped them to keep RA calm. You have a range of RA adapted exercises, even yoga which I do now. Also, regular walking, indoor cycling and swimming is very beneficial. Anything you do for at least 15 mins is so beneficial and pain friendly. If you do it a couple of times daily it's even better.

If you cannot motivate yourself easily, then apply for online courses and don't skip them. You simply need that for your wellbeing. All kinds of exercise, even simple for hands, can prevent quick joint damage. And you will feel good, speaking from my experience. I thought I couldn't do many yoga poses, but my yoga teacher helped me to figure out that I could. Little joints are extremely sensitive if not moving all the time, so use even stress balls for hand and fingers muscle strength. Remember: joint motion is a joint lotion, as many RA patients would say.

In the end, I would recommend staying positive and strong. This illness is hard, but still it can be put under control unlike some other worse diseases. If you are depressed, which is normal, don't forget to socialize and even go to psychotherapy too. Your mindset and feelings are also important and you need a lot of self-care to bring yourself into the balance. I realized that I needed to change my habits, attitudes and to love myself more. If I loved myself more earlier, maybe I wouldn't be disabled today.

Please focus on your health improvement on time and in the proper way, so your RA can be brought under control, I am sure. Hope you can learn from my example what you need to do in a very early phase.

Stay well and join the Instagram arthritis community, where you can exchange your condition and learn helpful tips from many other RA warriors.

Jane Bradley

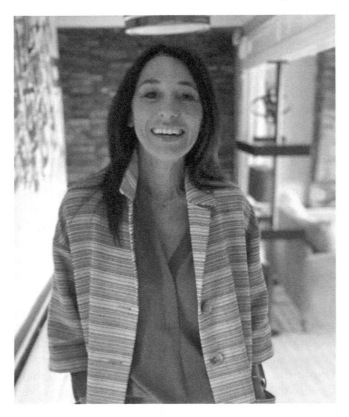

"The obstacles and journeys of living with rheumatoid."

For years I suffered with skin problems and digestive issues, then for well over a year joint problems. What I know now is,, sleeplessness, chronic pain that started in a finger, then kept moving, finally resulted in a diagnosis of rheumatoid arthritis in November 2019. Along with Raynaud's, osteoporosis and gastroesophageal reflux, RA spiraled quickly through my joints. I had a steroid injection and was put on methotrexate tablets, which made me so sick and caused worsening reflux. So I was changed to injections after 12 weeks with no improvement and hydroxychloroquine was then added.

Lockdown hit and made living with a chronic illness harder. My mouth problems started around now with a painful, dry sore coated tongue. I couldn't eat, I just drank water. I was battling so much my jaw started hurting and I had insomnia for months. After battling to see a consultant I was diagnosed with temporomandibular joint dysfunction, sicca complex and fibromyalgia. Yeah more to join the party. I was also put on baricitinib as my previous medication failed. I started getting used to this new med and more side effects but had no improvement. This impacted my mental health. All this time and before being diagnosed I was seeing a physio. She was amazing and could treat my jaw too, not a cure but relief. I had so many setbacks and obstacles. It never seemed to move forward, the chronic pain, continued painsomnia, more meds for evening pain causing more dry mouth, each also causing constipation so more drugs. I was then diagnosed with depression and anxiety by my GP and rheumatologist. My gp started ringing me every week in Nov 2020, then started adalimumab, known as humira injections, fortnightly alongside methotrexate.

By Christmas my pain was off the scale so I rang the rheumatology helpline, who I had previously rang a few times and came off the phone in tears. My own doctor said it's not helpful to be told they couldn't do anything, to basically get on with it. As it was my TMJ they could do nothing at this time as I was waiting to see a specialist for this and paying privately for help. By February I was on morphine as the pain in my head was so bad I could not put it on my pillow. Sinus problems, my throat, the list of illnesses was long and I felt like I really could not go on and didn't want to be here in this body. I had had enough, so between me and my gp we worked out it was the side effects of humira. She spoke to my rheumatologist and I came off it. It took 12 weeks to leave my body as did my side effects.

Each week got better thank God, but my rheumatoid got worse and was now in my jaw, elbows, ankles, knees and was so bad I was shuffling when I walked. My chronic pain got worse and fast forward to July 2021 I started my first infusion rituximab and was given steroids with it to alleviate some of the pain. I was so hopeful for something to work but started with worsening constipation. I contacted my nurse but it wasn't rituximab causing the issue. By September I was so bad I was admitted by my doctor to hospital for investigation. I was so severely constipated I looked nine months pregnant and was sick, as food had nowhere to go. It turned out I was severely blocked up so they gave me lots of medication to help.

My body had had enough and I fell in the garden (another set back). I had two spinous process fractures (broke my neck). I was lucky it was not too severe, I had a brace on my neck and could not move for six weeks. I also fractured my clavicle and suffered a right distal radius fracture, which after three weeks was not healing so I had surgery and a metal plate put in. It was another setback, so I didn't really get any relief from my rituximab and at Christmas 2021 it wore off.

Mid January I had my second round of rituximab for chronic pain from my jaw to my feet. I was just starting to come round and in March this year caught Covid. I was so ill I could not breath and was in hospital. I was offered sotrivamab, a neutralizing monoclonal antibody, which kills Covid. Thank God for medical research and life saving treatment. The joy of rituximab, it can't fight infections and I still had a secondary infection on my chest and needed strong antibiotics. Covid, tongue oral thrush, oral herpes, and then I had a massive flare, as I had come off my methotrexate for four weeks, so I was given a depo injection.

I started back on my methotrexate a couple weeks ago and now have the after effects of Covid and low mood depression. My gp has spoken or seen me now every Friday for over 18 months. She has kept me going and I share everything with her. She emails my rheumatologist with my problems that he needs to help me with and she helps with my other health problems that have come since being diagnosed with rheumatoid. I don't know where I'd be without her. I can't remember, since 2018, having no pain, no illness. My journey with RA has been complex with many obstacles. As well as physio and acupuncture, I have been doing yoga with @therayogi. She's the best yoga meditation instructor so it helps. I recently started swimming.

I haven't really thought about remission with so much going on for years. I just hope for the future, for a better quality of life. Definitely rituximab is doing that and hopefully I can start having more quality of life and enjoying the simple things after so many obstacles and challenges. My mouth will always be a problem which is hard and digestive problems are worse with the meds side effects. Living life, loving everything is important and I have the best husband of 30 years. I'm so blessed in many ways. Rheumatoid has changed my life in many ways but I've learned to be stronger in many ways so this year I can start enjoying life. I just wish people understood more about invisible illnesses. As they say never judge a book by its cover, I will keep raising awareness so we are understood better. Chronic pain is definitely misunderstood even by medical people too. Here's to battling life and spoonie love and support, I so appreciate love. Sleep has never been good since becoming ill. I've always been slim but I've lost more weight as I don't eat as well now with mouth problems. Mentally I can't concentrate the same and I am worse when flaring or in more pain. Forgetfulness and brain fog are not really mentioned by your rheumatologist but are awful. You can sometimes feel like you have dementia at times as it is so bad.

There are so many challenges for you and your body, after starting your journey with RA, that it is hard to deal with. Finding support online with others has so helped me for support and chatting and I would recommend it to anyone newly diagnosed. Never giving up is an option thouthough realize over the years that you don't know what each day will bring. That is why we are warriors. We keep fighting and not giving up. Enjoy the good days and battle the bad days. This disease ain't going away. Your goals and dreams in life may have changed but you do it, get up, dress up and never give up.

Lisa Leso

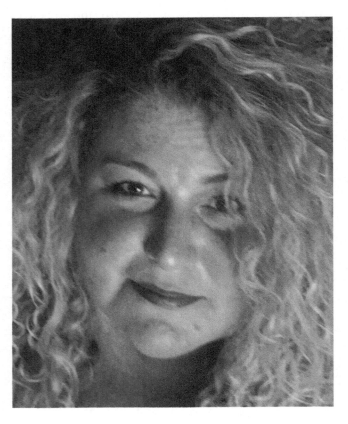

"A new normal."

It all started with just a swollen toe back in 2013. Within a year of seeing different doctors, I was officially diagnosed with psoriatic arthritis in 2014. I had never heard of the disease. I know I had suffered with psoriasis in the past but didn't know it could be a precursor to this! Since diagnosis I have had to adjust to a new normal life. I have decreased mobility and need an aid to walk (which can be difficult mentally with the stares I get). I needed to relearn to drive and was licensed with hand controls for my car after not being able to drive for two years. I have a handicapped placard as well. Most of my activities have to be planned out because of the pain. I have to alternate between standing and sitting because neither are comfortable for too long a time. My doctors have been able to somewhat control the pain by prescribing biologic meds (like you see in the TV commercials), shots every week of a low dose chemo drug and many pills and supplements.

I never in a million years thought I would feel pain head to toe in my 40s and now into my 50s! It is increasingly more difficult to exercise which has caused weight gain and affects the physical and mental side of this disease. The medications cause side effects which add more pills to that pill box and additional side effects of their own. There is also the "joy" of dealing with the insurances and authorizations to get the medications needed! Just adding to the roller coaster of stress which detrimentally affects my body. I have changed from working a full time schedule to a part time schedule, due to fatigue and pain. Yes...a lot has changed!

I have learned a lot about myself and my strength since this diagnosis. It has been an almost unbelievable road but I am thankful for the wonderful people at New Haven Rheumatology, my amazing family, friends and coworkers. I have met many wonderful online friends on Twitter and other arthritis sites, along with participating in the local arthritis walks. I am lucky and very fortunate to have a great support system.

Many people say to me, with all you go through in your life, how is it that you are always smiling? I don't really have an answer for that one, but no matter what happens in my life I always have faith and hope and always remember to count my blessings!

Love and hugs, Lisa

Caitlin Godfrey

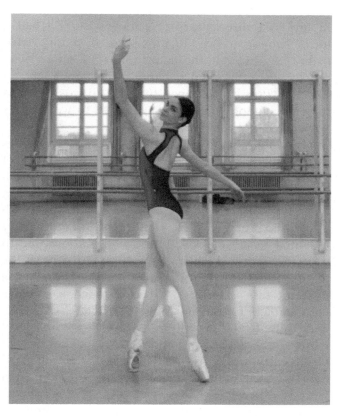

"The best part about hitting rock bottom, is that the only way is up!"

I have been diagnosed with enthesitis related arthritis (ERA), a type of juvenile idiopathic arthritis (JIA). I am in the midst of training to become a professional ballet dancer and wish to have a career in dance.

I began experiencing symptoms of arthritis in my feet about three years ago, but they were put down to dance training and they were treated like sports injuries. I was experiencing synovitis around my big toe joints and various other places in my feet. It wasn't until my symptoms spread to my elbows and wrists that my father, who is a physio, began to wonder whether it was more than just the high demands of ballet training.

He was correct. I began to see rheumatologists and it all pointed to arthritis. Eventually, I was diagnosed with ERA in the summer of 2021.

ERA is an autoimmune condition that causes pain and inflammation, at the point where ligaments and tendons attach to your bones.

People expected me to be devastated with the diagnosis because of the career path I have chosen, but to be brutally honest, I was relieved. I had spent so long wondering why I was getting these 'injuries' and no one else was, that it had started to frustrate me as it was hindering my ability to do what I love. So when I was confronted with ERA, and the correct treatment and medication was presented, it felt like a weight had been lifted from my shoulders.

Of course the diagnosis didn't stop the immense pain that I had been in. Some days I could barely walk, let alone dance but I was glad that I could see light at the end of the tunnel.

To start my treatment, I began with methotrexate injections. Unfortunately they didn't seem to have great effect, so I was also put on idacio injections. The combination seems to have worked wonders. It did take about six months to get the balance right, but my arthritis is settling now.

I have the possibility of going into remission some day and I hope it's on its way. The continued love and support of my family has allowed me to accept my chronic illness and face whatever it throws at me next.

I have found it is a lot easier to live with a chronic condition when you have someone to prop you up on your worst days.

I have also created an Instagram account, called Painfully Beautiful, to reach out and spread awareness of the chronic illness community.

Karol Silverstein

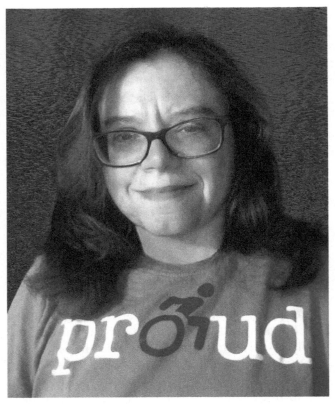

"What was I thinking?" I'd signed up for an undergraduate summer abroad program in Madrid and, as my departure neared, I was terrified. Newly disabled, I wasn't sure I could handle it. I went anyway."

Llamame MacGuyver

(aka call me MacGuyver)

"What was I thinking?"

This is what my brain was playing in an endless loop in the days leading up to my departure for an undergraduate summer program in Madrid. Sure, I'd handled a week-long trip to Madrid, with my college's Spanish Club the Christmas before, but this was six weeks, in a minimally structured program, living with a host family and taking hard classes.

I'd lived with my mom since crossing the threshold from having a chronic illness, due to a juvenile arthritis diagnosis at 13, to having a disability at 21. My disabled identity and navigating a world not designed for my disabled body were still fairly new to me. I'd done well, really well, in my first three years of college. But I'd had a lot of support along the way. Case in point, I still hadn't figured out the sock donner. I mean, why bother when my mom is happy to put my socks on for me? (Plus, I'd planned to move to Los Angeles for grad school, where I'd never need to wear socks anyway(or so I thought.)

It's not that I was against disability aides in general. I was a whiz with a dressing stick. I jokingly liken them to Batman's utility belt, which always seems to have the exact tool he needs in any given situation. The tasks I can handle with my trusty dressing stick are endless. I'm similarly indebted to my car key lever, which allows me to use gross motor skills, rather than fine motor skills, to turn over the ignition and magically makes a difficult task effortless. I'd also found a suitcase large enough to transport my toilet seat riser after a disastrous trial run with a "portable" version (quit while you're ahead on that one). I was all set, wasn't I? Actually, no. I was terrified. But, as with most terrifying challenges I face, I was going to do it anyway.

The director of the summer abroad program asked me what my needs for lodging were (my answer: first floor or a building with an elevator, within four or five blocks to the school, i.e. walking distance for me) and whether I wanted him to disclose my disability to the host family. To the latter, I said,"yes, absolutely." The last thing I wanted was to show up in Spain and be introduced to a host family that had no idea I was disabled. At the very least, it might be super awkward. At worst, perhaps they'd be ableist and so uncomfortable they'd back out.

After a bus trip from Philly to New York City and an overnight flight, I and the other students in the program arrived in Madrid, equal parts bleary-eyed and excited. The first thing on our agenda was a getting-to-know-one-another breakfast. I was more exhausted than hungry (I'd completely run out of spoons* somewhere over the Atlantic), but I soldiered through. At least the café con leche was strong as hell.

Finally, it was time to connect with our host families and be taken back to the homes we'd be staying in followed, immediately I hoped, by an opportunity to rest. As the group made its way to the meet up area, with me slowly bringing up the rear, the program director appeared beside me and quietly said, *"I decided not to disclose your disability after all."* Say WHAT?

He was afraid that people would shy away from hosting a disabled student for any number of reasons, ranging from liability concerns to outright ableism, and he was determined to accommodate my desire to participate in the program. He figured it'd be easier to navigate any potential fallout after the fact, and ultimately, I realized he had a point. People are sometimes weird around disability no matter how well you try to address their questions and concerns.

I didn't have much time to fret over the coming awkwardness anyway because, a minute later, I was being introduced to the woman who would house and feed me for the next six weeks. Her face registered the expected surprise. I am not someone with an "invisible disability." Among other tell-tale signs, I have significant hand deformities. To her credit, though, the surprise was merely a blip. The next challenge, I realized, would be communication. Turns out, my Spanish was not nearly as decent as I thought. Plus, she spoke no English and spoke Spanish muy rapido. Luckily arthritis is the same in both Spanish and English, just pronounced slightly differently, ar-THREE-teece, with those pesky i's sounding like long e's, so I was able to bring her up to speed on that at least.

Awkwardness over, we headed back to the woman's apartment, and she showed me the guest room (a roommate was to join me in another day). I let her know in my sub-decent Spanish that I needed to take a nap. I slept for nearly 12 hours. Seriously, she was worried about me.

When I finally did wake up, she offered me food and a shower. Then she gave me a key to the apartment and, through simple words and hand motions, I let her know I wanted to try locking and unlocking the door. Keys and locks were sometimes tricky for my hands. So much depends on angles. If a particular lock required an angle my hands weren't down for, I was in trouble. So, we did a test run. I took the key out into the hall, and she locked the door behind me. Deep breath. Insert key. Turn.

Except, it wouldn't turn. I tried leaning against the door, to apply pressure. No dice. Maybe pulling

out on the knob would help? Nope. I used my other hand. Both hands. Pulled up, down. All the while my host was shouting helpful suggestions through the door, which I couldn't really understand, but the concern in her voice matched my own. After struggling for about 15 minutes, she unlocked the door and let me back in the apartment. There was no verbal communication needed at this point because we were both thinking the same thing: What the hell were we going to do?!

I retreated to my room to think. Or maybe it was to hide. Or maybe to fall apart.

I tried to imagine how the six weeks ahead would possibly work without my having the freedom to come and go as needed. Would I have to wait outside the apartment door until my host got home to let me in? That seemed potentially unmanageable. What if I had to wait for hours? Was there even somewhere to sit? (I didn't remember seeing a chair in the lobby of the building). Maybe there's a friendly neighbor we could make arrangements with who'd unlock the door for me? That could mean lengthy waits as well, though.

I implored my adaptation-savvy brain to work its magic and then my car key popped into my mind, with its lever that turned a difficult, fine motor task into an easy, gross motor task. This was an instance where my inexperience as a traveler came in handy. I was an over-packer, like to a hysterical degree. I'd not only brought enough clothes for four months but a ridiculous amount of school supplies. Don't judge me, I just wasn't sure what I might need! I put the apartment key between two pens, positioning it at the end of the pens and at a slight angle. Then I secured it with masking tape, wrapping the entire length of pens completely for stability. I had my lever!

Emerging from my room, I managed to communicate to my host that I wanted to try the door again, showing her the gadget I'd made. She looked confused but, sensing my excitement, hopeful.

So again, I went out into the hall, and she locked the apartment door behind me…The door unlocked effortlessly.

Again, non verbal communication was necessary as we shared this moment of triumph, mixed with joy and relief, together. That was when I knew I'd be okay that summer—and beyond.

Cynthia Covert

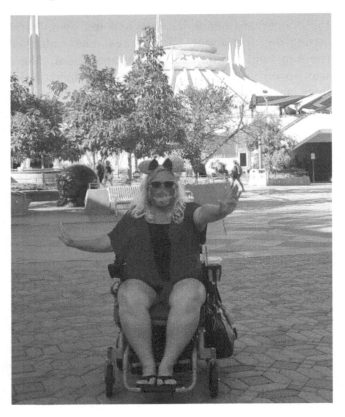

"Before my autoimmune arthritis diagnosis, I never envisioned mobility aids being a part of my life. My friends and I joked about a future of racing walkers or wheelchairs as senior citizens, but never gave serious thought to being dependent on one. Enter debilitating pain from multiple chronic illnesses."

Before my autoimmune arthritis diagnosis, I never envisioned mobility aids being a part of my life. My friends and I joked about a future of racing walkers or wheelchairs as senior citizens but never gave serious thought to being dependent on one. Enter debilitating pain from multiple chronic illnesses.

My life as a mobility aid user began a year after my fourth diagnosis. Within three years, I was diagnosed with psoriasis, psoriatic arthritis, fibromyalgia, and endometriosis. I have no idea what life would have been like with just one of them because symptoms for all were present long before the first one.

My first mobility aid was a manual wheelchair donated by the church I attended. I will never forget their generosity or the fact that they recognized that I was struggling long before I did. It was perfect for extended outings that required a lot of standing and walking. But it was too heavy for me to load and unload from our van. So after two years of avoiding shorter outings, I purchased my first rollator.

Using the rollator was a dream come true. It helped with balance and provided a place to rest when my feet or back needed to rest. However, at that time in my life, the only other people I saw using one were over 80 years old. There I was in my mid-thirties, feeling like I was living in an alternate universe. A universe in which I didn't feel like I fit in. Thankfully by my forties, the use of mobility aids for painful chronic conditions became more common. Seeing others in my age bracket using one validated my own need.

One of the reasons I was always hesitant to use a mobility aid was fearing that I would never know life without one. To my surprise, I began an alternative treatment in my late forties, and psoriatic arthritis responded exceptionally well to it. So well that I suddenly found myself going from using a manual wheelchair for all outings to using a rollator, crutches, and sometimes nothing at all. Tempted to donate or sell the mobility aids I no longer used, something told me to wait. Thankfully I did, because two years later I was back to using a wheelchair for every outing when my body stopped responding to the treatment. Part of me was disappointed, while another knew that the relief I was experiencing would not last.

Until this point, I had always struggled with the idea of needing to rely on mobility aids. But something changed during those two years of mobility freedom. I learned to appreciate the devices that had been there for me all those years and were still there to keep me moving after my body gave out. Instead, the hurdle I needed to conquer was one of not wanting to be reliant on others.

I had accepted my need for assistive devices, but I was not ready to let go of my independence. With arthritis damage progressing in my shoulders, elbows, and hands, getting around with a manual wheelchair required having someone to push me around. After a heartfelt talk with my husband, we agreed that a power wheelchair would be our next big investment. I say investment because a mobility aid is more than a purchase; we were investing in my health and life.

Life with a power wheelchair is better than I could have ever predicted. I am no longer stuck in a corner while waiting for my family to exit a ride at Disneyland. Instead, I am free to shop, go to a different attraction, or just hang out and people watch on Main Street.

My husband and children saw firsthand the pain that consumed me after outings without a mobility aid. They also benefited from my ability to do more at home after an outing with assistance. But my need for mobility devices hasn't always been accepted by those who do not live with me.

Not everyone was supportive. Some family and friends complained about trying to fit my wheelchair or rollator into their vehicles, or of the inconvenience of checking ahead to see if a place was accessible. Those who never had to rely on assistance suggested that purchasing a powered wheelchair was a waste of money, until they experienced an outing with me zipping around independently and saw firsthand the personal power it restored in me.

If I have learned anything in my 21 years of living with autoimmune arthritis, it is that having the right mobility aid can change your life. Having the right attitude makes it even better! Instead of viewing them as a means to an end, as in waiting until we cannot walk or stand, society should look at mobility aids as part of an effective pain management plan and preventative medicine.

My mobility aids do more than help me move. They help me end the day in less pain than if I didn't use one. Using a power wheelchair whenever I leave the house allows me to remain mobile at home. With psoriatic arthritis recently progressing into my hips and worsening in my knees, I am impressed that while at home, I only need occasional use of crutches and a walker.

When dealing with people who think arthritis patients who use mobility aids are lazy or giving in to their disease, I remind them that it is my life, not theirs. Because what I have noticed is that the ones who protest the most are actually projecting their own feelings. They are people who have never been in the position I am. At worst, they may have experienced a broken leg or foot, but their time of needing assistance was short-lived. They have no idea what it is like to live in a body that hurts all of the time and will never heal.

I share this portion of my story for two reasons. The first is to shine a light on the individual needs of arthritis patients. No timeline dictates when a person needs assistance from a mobility aid. And last but not least, to bring normalcy to the use of mobility aids within the arthritis community. The use of crutches, rollators, and wheelchairs should be accepted and not questioned by those who physically function without pain.

Sarah Dillingham

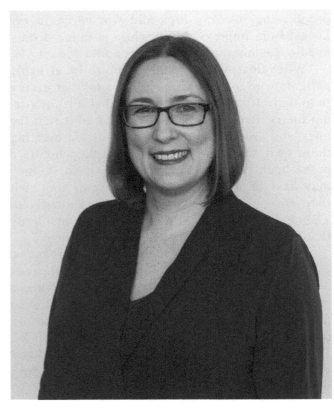

"Disability sneaks up on us when we're already in the middle of our lives, creeping into our careers, our families and social activities. Many of us benefit greatly from using adaptive aids like canes. They can help us to keep doing the things we love. So why is there so much stigma around using these devices? And why are we internalizing it?"

How I Learned To Rock A Cane In The Office

It was the third elevator that I'd attempted to call that day. I'd been stuck on a corporate landing for a good ten minutes, feeling panicky that I was late for my meeting.

There was nothing wrong with the elevators. They were arriving quickly. I was just too slow to get into them before the doors closed.

Rheumatoid disease (aka rheumatoid arthritis) had caused my feet and knees to swell up, leaving me in great pain.

Barely able to walk, I started thinking about getting a cane. I needed it for balance and stability. Maybe I could even use it to propel myself into the elevator in a timely fashion.

But the thought of bringing a cane into the office filled me with shame and anxiety. That's because so much of my corporate work life was dedicated to projecting a sense of professionalism and competence. Qualities that are not usually associated with disability.

Disability stereotypes tend to cluster at one of two extremes: the poor victim who needs to be looked after, or the inspirational hero. But that ignores the majority of us who are regular people living within unexpected limitations.

In the USA, arthritis is the leading cause of disability. According to the Centers of Disease Control and Prevention, arthritis affects 58 million people.

Disability sneaks up on us when we're already in the middle of our lives, creeping into our careers, our families, and social activities. Many of us benefit greatly from using adaptive aids like canes. They can help us to keep doing the things we love.

So why is there so much stigma around using these devices? And why are we internalizing it?

I didn't want to bring a cane to work because it signified frailty, decline, and weakness. Never mind that I was 36 years old, and needed it to stand up.

Instead, I continued shuffling around, strapping heat packs to my knees under my desk, and hoping that nobody would notice. Inevitably they did notice, which brought the concerned comments, quickly followed by the well-meaning questions.

That was swiftly followed by the unsolicited advice. Turmeric, yoga and cherry juice. It was clear that I couldn't hide my health condition and I couldn't stop people gossiping, so I adopted a new tactic.

I saw the opportunity when I joined a new team. On my first day, I sent out an introduction:

'I'm Sarah, I'm looking forward to working with you on this project. I have rheumatoid disease. It's a condition where my immune system attacks the soft tissues and joints in my body. My condition is well managed with the support of my rheumatologist. It does not affect my ability to do my job, although you may see me rocking a cane from time to time. If you have any questions, feel free to ask!'

Getting out in front of the gossip worked. People asked their questions in response to the email, and I didn't have to deal with the whispers and drip drip drip of curious stares. Instead, I discovered co-workers who would not only hold the lift for me, they'd kindly organize meetings on the floor I sat on so that I didn't have to walk too far.

I felt understood and respected which made it very easy for me to use the things I needed in the office - my cane, my compression gloves, and my beloved heat packs.

It's very hard to be vulnerable when you have chronic pain. So many of us feel the need to hide our conditions for fear of being judged or excluded. Disclosing disability in the workplace is a very personal decision and it's not right for everyone. I was fortunate to be met with empathy and understanding. This helped me to get past my own hang-ups around adaptive devices.

Now I see them as tools for personal freedom and use them with pride.

Therese Humphrey

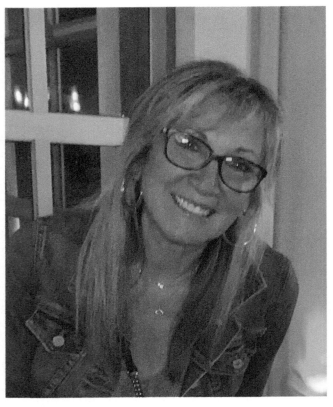

"It's never the tears that measure my pain, often it's the smile I fake!" My life with rheumatoid arthritis."

It's difficult for me to stay brief about 36 years living with rheumatoid arthritis with the many highs and lows. I was diagnosed in 1986 at age 25. There is no doubt this is one hard ass disease BUT when you are able to find "that treatment" that works for you, to stop the progression, you CAN start living a little bit better again, if not a whole lot better!

Today in 2022, I think of all these past years and the challenges I have endured and persevered. Over time, I have learned and still continue to learn so much about myself. The real strength I knew I had, but I just had to find it as I was met with many challenges to overcome.

RA has taught me a lot about personal strength, a stronger empathy toward others and never giving up hope for better days. Even now, I still have days I struggle and days I curse that I've been stricken with this body destroying disease. It's taken away my career as a registered nurse. Yes, I still grieve on any given day but I know I have no other choice but to accept my limitations and move on. I have found the courage to let go of what I cannot change, so that I can continue moving forward and enjoy the best life has to offer.

That is what RA brings, a 24hr day to day disease, that has tons of systemic symptoms that are unpredictable and some that can be predictable. I consider this disease as a "blood disease" affecting the immune system and is not solely a joint disease. It affects the entire body and luckily, at this point, I do not have any organ damage. I work closely with my rheumatologist, every three to four months with checkups and blood tests to make sure I stay in control along with my current treatment.

On my good days of less pain, I embrace the things that I am able to do. Brushing my teeth, blow drying my hair, lifting a coffee cup, walking, bending, functioning without excruciating pain. It's those littlest of things that I never take for granted.

In 1986, at age 25, my RA diagnosis came at a time when no medications were available that stopped the progression. Within an eight year period I became disabled. During the several years from diagnosis, RA's progression caused fusion of my wrists and ankle bones causing no range of motion. The synovial fluid is gone and bones literally grew/fused together over a short period of time.

In 1998/1999, my rheumatologist enrolled me in a new "RA" drug trial *now known as Enbrel, *the first Biological medication. After this trial, I was placed on this new anti-TNF biologic, enbrel, which finally stopped the advanced destruction that RAwas causing. My pain decreased and after 3 months, I was considered in a "drug induced" remission.

The biggest loss I have encountered that hasn't been physical, is losing friends. Friends that could not understand my "mask" of a smile I wore everyday, despite the pain and fatigue that my disease caused. I truly feel my positive upbeat attitude was a blessing for me getting through all those years, yet a curse, having the ignorance of friends not truly understanding the "invisible" aspect of this horrific disease. It's hard and still today continues to be, which is why I try my best to explain all that RA brings to anyone that's willing to listen.

Since that time, I encountered a huge setback in 2016, with RA striking its ugly head again, causing me to be almost bedridden with extreme fatigue and inflamed joints. I struggled and changed biological medication several times over that one and a half years of constant flaring, as recommended by my rheumatologist.

I did my own research at the time too, wondering why my medication failed. Was there a possible "trigger" that caused my decline and not the medication losing efficacy!?

So, I decided to do some research of my own, given I was aging, I looked up online various studies (on reputable sites) and found several research studies on low hormone levels worsening RA. This made me want to take a closer look at myself, knowing that I was at the menopausal age. Could this be the cause of my RA worsening and not the biologic medication failing?

My hormone levels revealed exactly that, definitive menopause. I decided after much research and discussion with my gynecologist to start a bioidentical hormone replacement therapy. Within three weeks, I started feeling better with lessening in fatigue as well as joint inflammation. I truly feel at that time, that it was my hormone replacement therapy that may have been the answer all along, and not that the biologic stopped working. I ended up going back to taking the original biologic,(anti-TNF) in 2018, and continue with positive results today.

From 2011 to 2020, I have had several surgical arthrodesis procedures on both feet, toes, ankle and a total left knee replacement. This was all due to erosion and damage from RA prior to remission. I am currently in need of the other ankle to be surgically fused, to help lessen the pain and strengthen the joint.

Chronic pain has become my "norm." My symptoms fluctuate and can be aggravated by too much activity or not enough. Walking or standing for long periods of time is what I try to avoid. I have learned and try to keep control by taking extra care/precautions that I know can aggravate my symptoms. I use a mobile scooter to avoid the possible "aftermath" of pushing myself by walking too far. It was the best investment I have made.

RA is without a doubt a cruel, unforgiving, debilitating disease when not treated and controlled. After 36 yrs, it has left its mark on me, leaving joint destruction and damage, causing loss of function, disability and chronic pain in varying degrees every single day.

It is okay to say to yourself, "it can always be worse." This can be very productive. However, saying it to someone else can dismiss what they are going through but saying it to yourself, certainly helps me with my mindset to deal with the pain and getting through the worst of days.

My limitations and chronic pain leave me with only focusing on modifying everything I do to prevent increasing pain. I fight everyday that never ending fear of what "could" be, but I try to turn that fear around and focus on the things in life that are in my control: my mindset, my happiness, modifying and acknowledging all that I am able to do.

My love and passion for exercise along with effective medications (biologics) and a healthy anti-inflammatory diet, has made me able to cope and manage a little bit better. Exercising has always made me feel like I have some control. I believe I have held onto some of my muscle strength that I probably would have lost a long time ago!

I will never let this disease take my spirit no matter how hard it tries. I will never give up "Hope." After all these years, I've lived a life of hope. I'll continue to hope for good days, hope for better days, hope for a cure!

Janet Plank

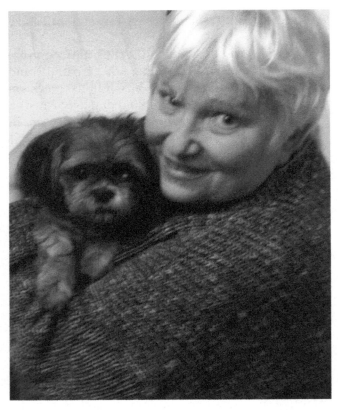

"The right knee, I put off for a later date. I haven't had surgery on that right knee yet. I am overweight and truly believe that losing weight will make a difference in my joints, with or without surgery. To date, I have lost 38 pounds and have a long way to go, however, I do notice a difference."

It Began With a House Call

Way back in the late 1950s, and early 1960s, doctors made house calls. Back pain in an active child can be debilitating. The next thing I knew, I had to take my shirt and pants off, leaving my panties on. Onto the table I climbed and rolled over to my stomach. My mom was there, and I am guessing my grandma. With both my mom and my dad gone, I can't get details anymore. The doctor passed away years ago.

He thought I had scoliosis. There was so much back pain. Then, to the hospital for x-rays. I am fairly certain that an x-ray machine ruled out scoliosis.

We trusted our doctors to diagnose and treat us. However, I don't know how accurate testing was back then.

That pain still exists in my back, my spine. My neck as well. Physical therapy has been an off-and-on-again part of my life from childhood through adulthood.

Have you heard of growing pains? Did you have them?

That pain is something else I experienced when I was young. That pain was with me for a long time. I remember the pain in my tibia bones. Nothing hurt that bad. I remember crying because of the extreme pain. I couldn't sleep. It seems that I was quite active during the day. Back then, someone said it was a form of arthritis.

Looking up growing pains on the Mayo Clinic's website it says: *"it's an ache or a throb in the legs, often in the front of the thighs, the calves or behind the knees. They tend to affect both legs and they occur at night."* I just remember the pain in my bones.

Now I have severe joint and muscular pains.

My mid 30s brought me to another adventure and the first time anyone mentioned osteoarthritis.

Working on the second floor and having a two-story house lost its appeal big time. The steps were getting tough. My left knee started hurting. Thinking that I needed more exercise or even stretches, I did them. The pain increased. Then, the clicking started. Soon after, my knee would catch in the bent position. This sometimes happened even when walking. Mainly on the steps.

It was time for the doctor, before I went head-first down the steps, breaking something. I was scheduled to see an orthopedic surgeon. He was a great doctor, asked good questions, and gave good answers. I was impressed.

After my arthroscopy of the knee, there are three little scars on my left knee where the doctor scraped that arthritis away. Physical therapy went well. On my bottom, I scooted up and down the long flight of steps until I felt safe walking.

The doctor said that people with knees like mine usually belong to an older person, who winters in Florida. I really liked him.

That surgery was amazing. My knee felt 98% better. The only complaint that I had is that the cold was still so painful. If I had to be outside, I would wrap something around my knee for protection.

My back just wasn't going to stop hurting. I had physical therapy, injections, epidurals and back braces over the years. The pain gets relentless and over the top. I often wear sweatpants and sweatshirts, especially in the summer air conditioning, and the South Dakota winters.

Fishing was a favorite thing for my hubby, my dad, and myself. We were out in the boat. My dad had a nice fish on. I grabbed the net to bring in the fish. Leaning across the back of the boat, I started to reach out with the net and froze. My back... the pain was horrific. I couldn't help the tears that followed. My husband and dad both acted as if I lost it. Finally, I could respond, *"My back, my back!"*

I took Advil, and we made our 2 ½ hour trip home.

My doctor scheduled me with a neurosurgeon. He fused my L5 and S1 disks. There is the likelihood that I will be having additional surgeries down the road.

That surgery was such a blessing. I was surprised it felt so good. I'm not sure of the total recovery time frame after surgery, I just know it was amazing.

Now, what to do with the rest of my body.

- The orthopedic doc asked: *"Where is the pain?"*
- Me: *"everywhere!"*
- He said: *"we can't x-ray everything! So, pick a few places now and then we can add others on the next visit. Choose your two most painful and least controlled areas."*
- My reply: *"That's fine."* He took x-rays of my shoulder, hips, and knees. My shoulders and hips have bursitis. Both knees had arthritis.

My next appointment was with the orthopedic surgeons. Findings at my next appointments:

- **Feet with the lower joint surgeon:** Both feet need to have bones fused. Four on the right, some on the left. One foot at a time. The right first, with a month in a wheelchair, a month with a walker, and a month with a cane. Then, depending on how I'm getting along, we will do another foot. I told him I would call back to schedule. The doctor recommended shoes that I should be wearing and called the shoe store to let them know I would be stopping by after I left this appointment. I chickened out on foot surgery. I was afraid that my feet wouldn't heal as they were supposed to.

- **The hand surgeon:** Both hands are painful and arthritic. If the air conditioning was on or if I was out in the cold, I had to wear gloves. Before we could do anything, I needed neurological testing to see if I had carpal tunnel. Thankfully no. First a right thumb CMC arthroplasty, then the left thumb, CMC arthroplasty with FCR to APL tendon transfer. What a difference those surgeries made. Occupational therapy followed. The air conditioning still bothers my hands and arms. Thankfully the thumbs aren't an issue anymore.

- **My left total knee replacement was so needed and a huge success.** Physical therapy helped. It became apparent that I had been favoring my left leg and knee. It affected my back and whole posture.

- **The right knee, I put off for a later date.** I haven't had surgery on that right knee yet. I am overweight and truly believe that losing weight will make a difference in my joints, with or without surgery. To date, I have lost 38 pounds and have a long way to go, however, I do notice a difference.

- **My back and neck are the biggest pains.** I have fibromyalgia too, so I know it adds to the problem. Between the two, I'm in constant pain. I can only sit for so long, then I'm up for a while. It's wonderful that I'm able to be up more often. Losing weight has made a difference. After a while though, I recline in my adjustable bed, where I can still read and write. This does help my back feel better. Never will I lay for more than an hour, without getting up and moving around. My dogs do encourage exercise and playtime too. I do get up during the night to use the bathroom, so I take time to stretch and move around. It helps me sleep through the rest of the night.

• **A good mattress is so important.** Mattresses do affect every joint and muscle that I have.

I'm a firm believer that if you don't use it, you lose it. Plus, these joints stiffen up and get so painful. If you are obese or need to lose weight, this is a great time to do so. Talk to your doctor and/or nutritionist about the foods and diet you should follow.

• Do maintain exercise. Your doctor or physical therapist can advise.
• Only take medication prescribed by your doctor. Over-the-counter medications should be limited. They can cause as much harm as prescriptions and must be taken as directed. Discuss this and all medications with your doctors. It's important to know that they are compatible as well. At a time when medication is frowned upon, some people feel as if they are left hanging without options and with severe pain. Talk with your doctor about the course of action that you should follow and the choices that need to be made.
• For pain, alternating ice and heat packs might help you as well.

Pain, especially chronic pain can affect a person's mental or emotional state. This doesn't mean that you are crazy, it means that it can affect your mental health. I have trouble concentrating and focusing when I'm struggling with stabbing pain. Pain might affect you differently.

This is also part of your health. Your overall health.

Ray Bouchard

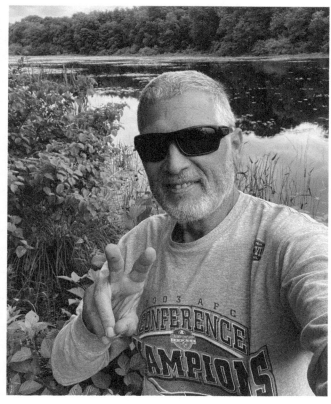

"Nothing mentioned here is a cure. There isn't one, I will not be a victim. I will not be seen as a victim. I understand it, I have a plan."

I am 68 and I have ankylosing spondylitis, rheumatoid and osteoarthritis. I am not a writer but people sharing in this community have helped me and it expands everyone's perspectives. I was diagnosed with seronegative rheumatoid arthritis in 2016. I was 62 years old. Over the next three years I tried/failed four biologics and three disease modifiers, I lost my job/career, I lost my identity and my RA was still unchecked. Listening to well-meaning doctors I had physically deteriorated and worse, I ballooned to three hundred plus pounds. Three years of high dose prednisone kept me alive, but I was huge and had trouble moving without a device.

I had my left hip replaced in that May and then in June I tried a new cocktail of drugs, methotrexate and humira and they worked, and I was able to significantly reduce prednisone from 280 mg to 30 mg per day, I got stuck there for a year and a half because my body was not producing enough corticosteroid during stress, so it took that long to taper to zero. It has been almost three years without prednisone.

I started following people who looked at problems differently. Now I am focused on just moving forward and feeling as good as I can in any given moment despite arthritis.

I am convinced that something environmental triggered my autoimmune system, to think attacking me was the best way to protect me. As a firefighter/first responder I was exposed to a list of chemicals that were not "yet" classified as toxic, atomized metals and concrete, plus the stress . I started to understand how some food was inflammatory and some was anti-inflammatory. I was spending $727 a month for humira and mostly everything I ate, drank, did and used, had the potential to cause inflammation. I needed to at least change something.

Over the past three years I have changed how I eat. It started with gluten. Do not eat gluten, then dairy and gradually I transitioned to eating mostly plant-based foods prepared by me, and I drink a lot of high-quality H2O. These changes helped significantly lessen inflammation, allowing me to reach remission for several months and, against my rheumatologist's advice, I have discontinued humira, and methotrexate and so far, my disease activity has been mild. Another benefit was being able to actually watch the improvement in my cardiac health. With my cardiologist's approval I was able to discontinue two heart medications, the first time he has recommended a patient to reduce med's.

This is not meant to be advice, it is my story. If you follow me on Instagram, you know I post my activities daily. I have found some things that work for me, the information is everywhere. I do not like diet labels, vegan, vegetarian, pescatarian, they do not hang well on me. I just try to eat food that is anti-inflammatory, gives me energy, is easy on my gut and helps with some of the myriad of morbidities and comorbidities that comes with RA, AS and OA. Thanks to eating differently and moving every day I have been able to claw back parts of my life, lose a lot of weight, and regain some confidence.

I would still run or at the least walk amazingly fast into a burning building for you. I am a firefighter. It is a part of me. It is "who" I am. I have arthritis. It's a group of very serious diseases. Nothing mentioned here is a cure. There isn't one. I will not be a victim. I will not be seen as a victim. I understand it, I have a plan.

Thank you so much for reading, hope the rest of your day is great.

Archie Hindle

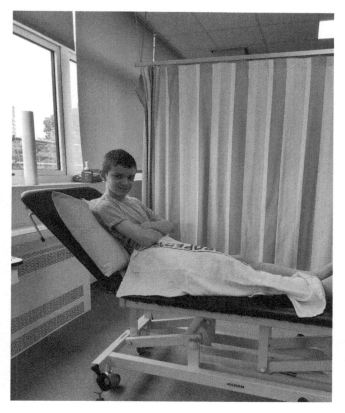

"I'm a JIA warrior."

I'm a warrior of JIA. I was diagnosed in December 2018 at the age of just eight, but I do think I had it longer as my legs have always hurt, I just didn't tell anyone. JIA affects both my ankles, knees and wrists and some days I find it extremely difficult to walk. Me and my family have been told I have 10° deformation of my left leg, but physiotherapy is slowly working in helping me straighten my leg out but it's so hard to do the exercises three times a day as my legs get tired. I also have to wear a splint in bed to help keep my leg straight while I sleep. Some days I'm not able to join in with PE at school. It upsets me to see my friends running about and playing football and I'm having to sit on the sideline because my legs are hurting and I'm not able to bend them. I find it the most difficult when me and my siblings are playing out in the garden and I'm not able to bounce on the trampoline as high as them, as it hurts my knees and ankles.

I push myself everyday to try and be like everyone else, but then the next day I'm suffering with pains in both my legs and ankles. It really hurts when I'm having a flare, my joints swell up, go red and get really hot. The pain is so bad that normal paracetamol and ibuprofen don't take the pain away. The only thing that helps me is having nice warm baths, but my mum and dad have to help me get up and downstairs which is a little embarrassing as I'm now 12 years old. I have to take 5 ml. of sulfasalazine twice daily and it doesn't taste nice at all and it's bright yellow. I also have to have adalimumab needles every two weeks, that really stings. I have to see my Rheumatology Nurse, Sam every three months and have my bloods taken every three months. I also see physiotherapy every three months with Abby. She's worried about my spine now, so I'm having extra checks on that when I see her.

But, like I said, I'm a JIA warrior and I'm NOT going to let this disability define me, even if I don't go into medical remission. I will try my hardest every single day to achieve my best and everyday I'm slowly working myself up to attending PE again.

Tammy Maltais

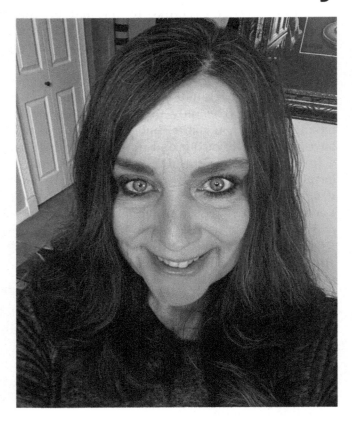

really listened to what I was experiencing. Since I was sick, the focus was on the other issues I had but not the horrific pain I was experiencing. After many tests this wonderful doctor said I was testing positive for RA and other autoimmune markers. I was sent to a rheumatologist in Denver where I was put on medication so they could get my RA under control.

As I look back, each day I'm thankful I made it through all the challenges I have faced. I was in a wheelchair for three years and had to learn how to walk again. Depression hit as each day I looked in the mirror, I would see how much hair and weight I had lost. I knew if I was to get better I had to push myself to get stronger. It took me two years to get where I am today but keeping positive and accepting of my diagnoses, helped me get my life back. To my fellow RA warriors, never give up, you can do it!

"The journey you take is yours to choose. Love yourself and take one day at a time to get where you want to go. Nothing is impossible!"

Five years ago I started my journey of health issues I never experienced before. I had just turned 49 and was thriving in my current career. I traveled a lot with my job and the demands of my job kept me busy, so I didn't notice the early symptoms I was experiencing. Within a few months my health had declined and the start of a nightmare began. It started in 2017 with several hospital stays, surgeries, and the most excruciating pain I had never dealt with before. I had a difficult recovery from all the surgeries as it took a toll on my body. In 2018, I was blessed with two drs that sat down with me in the hospital and

Jessie Riojas

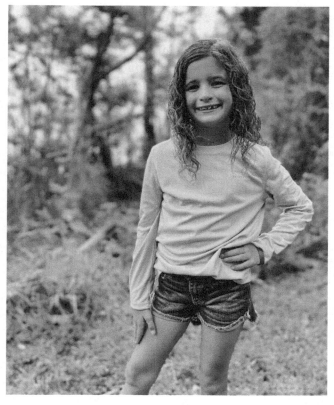

"Don't Stop Believing...In A Cure!"

This is Jessie's Journey...Jessie Riojas, age eight, has always been a very happy and active child. She has always kept her mom and dad on their toes. She has been active in swimming, since the early age of 18 months and gymnastics, since the age of two. In January of 2017, when Jessie was just three, her father and mother noticed her right knee starting to swell and by the end of February 2017, it was noticeably larger than her left knee (about two times the normal size). One morning in early March 2017, Jess had trouble getting out of bed and walking down the hallway. This was something that Jessie usually did at top speed every morning but this particular morning, Jessie used the wainscotting trim to help her get where she wanted to go. It was then that her parents, Mark and Jacquie Riojas, knew something serious was going on.

They contacted her pediatrician and were told to bring Jess in as soon as possible. The next couple of weeks were full of doctor appointments, exams, tests and labs. On April 3, 2017, Jessie was given the diagnosis of juvenile rheumatoid arthritis. Juvenile rheumatoid arthritis? What is that? Juvenile rheumatoid arthritis (or JRA for short), affecting approximately 300,000 kids in the US, can cause the immune system to mistake healthy cells and tissues as foreign substances, causing inflammation. The disease ranges in severity and can lead to not only serious joint issues but also uveitis, a dangerous inflammation of the eyes that can cause blindness. There is currently no cure but there are medications that help reduce symptoms. After consulting with their rheumatologist, Jessie was given a series of steroid injections, in hopes to get the inflammation under control, without having to begin other types of medication. After two rounds of steroid injections, unfortunately the inflammation was still there. It was after the steroid injections that Jess began multiple medications to help control the inflammation, including three different types of eye drops, four times a day, because she was also diagnosed with uveitis. Despite Jessie being on so many different types of medication for her arthritis, she never skipped a beat, remaining so positive and active during such a trying time. What a little warrior she was!

In August of 2020, after being on medications for more than three years, Jess was pronounced in remission and was able to come off of all medications. Although Jessie was in remission, it did not guarantee another flare up from occurring. In May of 2021, Jess yet again received the news that she was in another flare with JRA. This time the arthritis was back, in both of her knees as well as her eyes, causing swelling and inflammation once again. She was immediately put back on medication for both. As of today, February 9, 2022, Jessie is in medication remission. This means that there is no sign of active arthritis but she is still currently taking daily/weekly medications to help keep the arthritis under control. This has been a long and winding road but through it all, Jessie continues to smile. She is still involved in gymnastics and loves to swim. She also plays basketball and runs three miles with her dad any chance that they get.

Jess is an eight year old JRA warrior. Her family prays daily for a cure for JRA but until then, they will continue to fight and spread awareness of juvenile rheumatoid arthritis. Don't Stop Believing...In A Cure!

Valerie Bachinsky

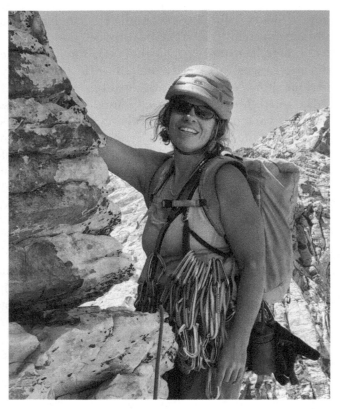

"Using My Osteoarthritis Journey to Help Others."

At the age of 48, I am happy to say that I am at the peak of my fitness and performing at a level I never dreamed possible. Yet, I have lived with osteoarthritis for over 20 years. During those 20 plus years, I have experienced plenty of setbacks and challenges, including times I feared my active life was over. But ultimately, I refused to give into my diagnosis and now use what I have learned to help others determined to fight their osteoarthritis. This is my story.

I was diagnosed with osteoarthritis in both knees when I was just 27. My doctor, at the time, gave me no advice other than "learn to put your feet up and relax." I could not believe what she had said to me and refused to believe I had to stop living the way I wanted to live. I had just started to develop a passion for the outdoors and a deep appreciation for nature. I was on my way to becoming an avid backpacker and was not ready to surrender the luscious sense of freedom I felt during long walks in the wilderness. I rejected the doctor's advice and continued to live life on my terms.

Knee pain simply became a part of my life. I remember occasionally having to wrap my knee up in duct tape to make it through a hike. I often lagged behind others, especially on descents which hurt my knees and feet. I simply did what I had to do out of love for what I was doing. I was still able to make progress with my hiking and dreamed of bigger mountains. I summited Mt. Baker in the Cascade Mountains, which was quite an accomplishment. The highlight of the trip however, was discovering rock climbing.

I felt like I had been waiting my whole life to rock climb and immediately fell in love. The sport is the perfect blend of mental and physical challenge, while also offering a sense of zen. I loved the movement, overcoming fear and the laser-focus it required. It soon took over everything else.

Around the same time, one of my knees became extremely irritated after wearing some not-too-high-heeled shoes. For months, my knee audibly knocked and descending steep hills became very painful. Sadly, I had to cancel a dream backpack trip in the Sierra mountains. It was the first time I had to cancel something because of my osteoarthritis. I was crushed.

Fortunately, my knee still allowed me to rock climb and the trip turned into an opportunity to learn more rock climbing skills. Or perhaps it wasn't so fortunate. The new skills I took back home with me may have produced a sense of overconfidence, which may have caused me to overestimate my ability. Once back home, I fell 20 feet while climbing. My ankle shattered. I had to be airlifted out of the wilderness by helicopter. It was a life changing injury in many ways. The surgeon told me I would never have a normal ankle again. In addition to the fracture, I lost a lot of ankle cartilage and suffered nerve and blood vessel damage. The nerve damage resulted in a contractured foot. Osteoarthritis developed in my ankle and foot soon after the injury. I would never regain full range of motion in the ankle and to this day it remains in a semi-fused state.

I was out of work for over two years and never able to return to the type of work I did as a hospital floor nurse again.

It wasn't all bad though. After the initial shock of the injury, I entered a period of self-discovery. I learned how to better care for myself. I discovered what it was like to be a patient, which led me to develop a high level of compassion that I did not possess before. This made me a better nurse.

I also discovered the gaps that existed in the healthcare system. Different providers fixed different parts but there was nothing in place to help me return to the whole person that I was prior to the accident. I became inspired to try to fill this gap.

I enrolled in an online college and pursued a degree in health education. It was my dream to become a health coach and educator, to help people achieve their highest level of wellness, after experiencing a setback like mine.

I eventually returned to work part-time as an employee health nurse. Although it was initially difficult to assume a new nursing role, eventually it became a very comfortable job. It was the perfect mix of sitting and standing that worked very well with my limitations.

I resumed rock climbing. I was extremely tentative and fearful at first but eventually returned to the fervor and passion that I had prior to the accident. However, now I have wisdom and a dedication to safety. Unfortunately, I was plagued with frequent injuries that would keep me off the rock from time to time. I would tweak one knee or the other, then a shoulder, next a foot. I always seemed to have some sort of joint problem or inflammatory injury. As a result, I couldn't reach the momentum I needed to improve, but I learned to be satisfied with what I could achieve.

Eventually, I continued on to earn my master's degree in nursing. This was a game changer for me both professionally and personally. Once done with my degree, I decided to move to Las Vegas due to its ease of climbing access and weather that allowed year-round rock climbing.

Life in Vegas did not initially go as planned. The move went well and I was quickly able to get a well-paying job. However, the job's environment was toxic and was very demanding. It began to take a mental and physical toll on me.

Then, Covid hit. My work load nearly doubled. The stress was debilitating. I had no time to care for myself and was rapidly gaining weight. My health and joints suffered. Finally, I decided to leave the position. As someone with a deep-seeded fear of financial insecurity, it was an extremely difficult decision. However, I was more fearful of my climbing dreams slipping away.

I was despondent and unsure of my future after leaving the job. It took several months for me to mentally recover from the stress. I toyed around with different ideas and then rediscovered my dream from years before. I began studying for a health coach certification.

I took a long-planned trip to the Sierra Mountains with the intention of hiking to and climbing Cathedral Peak, a long-time dream of mine. But the arthritis in my knee had advanced to the point that it would lock up and hiking had become painful. Once again, I found myself in my beloved Sierra Mountains, unable to achieve a dream objective because of my osteoarthritis. I felt as if I had hit a rock bottom with my OA.

I returned home determined to beat it.

I put my master's degree to work for me. I combed through the scientific literature looking for knowledge about what contributes to joint pain and degeneration. I discovered a ton of new research done on osteoarthritis in the past 20 years. Additionally, I sought information on motivation and emotions because I was very aware of how difficult it is to change health behaviors. I knew this journey had to start with learning to prioritize my health needs.

I designed and adopted a lifestyle intended to fight inflammation and reduce joint pain. I lost 50 pounds while also paying attention to all the other factors that affect osteoarthritis symptoms. I began to feel better than I had in 20 years. Most of my joint pain and susceptibility to injury vanished over time. I started to climb harder than I ever have. My dreams finally began to come true.

I also gained clarity on what I wanted to do with my life. I started a coaching business, focused on helping other women with osteoarthritis adopt and maintain a lifestyle that allows them to live their best life. I named it Genuine Glow Wellness, after my love for the way mountains glow in the early morning.

Through my work, I discovered that many myths and misconceptions still surround osteoarthritis. Many people are still told that little can be done to improve their OA, leading to feelings of hopelessness and confusion. It is now my mission to reach others to let them know that osteoarthritis is not a terminal diagnosis and much can be done to reduce OA symptoms and slow the progression.

It is so fulfilling to be making a positive impact in the lives of people who live with osteoarthritis like me. It seems that all the twists and turns of my life journey has led me to find my true passion of helping other people achieve the best possible version of themself.

Maddison Bevel

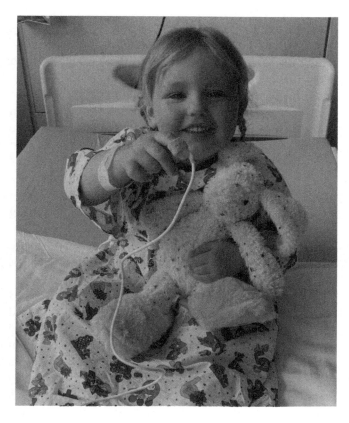

"It could be worse."

This is the one thing that gets me through everything. I'm so grateful that Maddison is here strong and plowing through.

Maddison was diagnosed in March 2020. Just after her first birthday in October, we noticed one day she stopped weight bearing and then completely stopped walking altogether. Maddison was hospitalized and was an outpatient and having IV antibiotics for six weeks before they could diagnose her with JIA, as no one was really sure what was wrong with Mads. She was sent to St. Thomas's, who did more tests, as Maddison symptoms led down two paths, leukemia and JIA. After a few weeks of discomfort for Mads and worry for us, she was diagnosed with JIA and started treatment straight away. She had to have a steroid operation in her ankle joint and both knees to help her walk and a weekly methotrexate injection that we were trained to do at home.

Like everyone we were hit with the Covid pandemic, but we're so grateful to be able to be at home at this time, to look after Maddison, as much as we could. James, my husband, built Mads a walker to help her learn to walk again after her op and we couldn't believe our eyes! A goodnight sleep and the next day she took her first steps! Before we knew it Mads was walking around on her own just a few months later! Maddison couldn't really walk a far distance and her injections made her feel a bit sick a few days after having them, but it was helping her mobility and that's what we were so grateful for! The blood tests that we had to have every three Months were tricky and not fun, but we had to just get on with it and it became part of Maddison's life. Maddison stayed in remission for two years and didn't relapse once! She came off her meds in March 2022 but shortly after, in May 2022, unfortunately relapsed. Not only did it affect her joints this time, it also affected her eyesight this was when things became more tricky for us as she had to go on six steroid eye drops a day which Maddison hated! She also had to have the steroid operation again.

It has been two weeks since Mads had her op and she's running around like she has new legs! She struggles with distance but is doing amazing. She's such a strong little girl. I know she will overcome all of this one day. We just have to push through this all for now.

Katie Simons

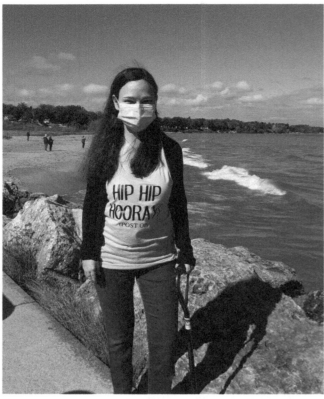

"Experiences and advice from a post-op hip replacement patient."

Hip Hip Hooray!
What I Now Know About Hip Surgery

Age matters. First thing I discovered was that my age was going to be an issue, which at the time was 30. My surgeon's office would call a week before my appointment, confirm details like my name, reason for the visit, the usual. But once they heard my date of birth, inevitably I would be put on hold, then rescheduled. The people answering the phone would not listen to anything after that. Even my rheumatologist couldn't get through to them. By the time I started the process for surgery it was about ten years after my rheumatologist told me hip replacement surgery would be in my future. By the time I actually saw the surgeon I was rescheduled about ten times. The time it took before I had the surgery was about ten months. So now, I urge anyone in a similar situation to at least make an appointment as soon as they can. On the other hand, luckily my age did make recovery easier and quicker for me.

There is a lot of cleaning. Protocols may differ between hospitals and surgeons. For me the week leading up to surgery was filled with cleaning. They instructed me to wear clean clothes every day, which is normal enough, but also clean bedding every night. That required a lot of extra laundry, and a lot of extra physical effort every day, all while being off my normal medications. I was also given special soap to use in the shower, that needed to be on my skin for five minutes before rinsing and no other cleansers, besides shampoo and conditioner. I had a physical therapist once recommend using the heat from a shower to help stretch, so I used that time for some gentle stretching instead of spending five minutes stressing about the procedure. And the next time I have surgery I will treat myself to some delightfully fragrant hair care products to use and enjoy.

Perspective matters. I would tell people that I was "eagerly dreading" my surgery. I knew I would feel better after, but it was still a daunting task. So instead of thinking of it as being strapped down naked and unconscious in a room full of strangers whose job it is to violently cut me open, I choose to think about it as a very bizarre spa day. Everyone's job was to make sure I was taken care of, to receive the care I needed to get better and healthier.

Have a pain plan. A lot of people were eager to give me drugs and to tell me to use them before I needed them. Only one nurse talked to me about not using the pain pills. That advice was invaluable. What I ended up doing was to always wait a little bit longer between each pill. A built-in tapering plan with the flexibility to ensure my pain was controlled for physical therapy appointments. That worked for me but be sure to talk to your health care team about your own needs. Plus ice packs, I used lots and lots of ice packs!

Celebrate it. I am not talking about some lavish party. But I wanted something to look forward to. So, I ordered an ice cream cake with "Hip hip hooray" written on top to enjoy once I got home. The night before my operation my mom also painted my toenails in the most glittery polish I had. Not only were these things something to look forward to, but it was fun and joyous. I had to be looking down while using a walker, but there was still some sparkle to keep me going.

Annastasha Parker

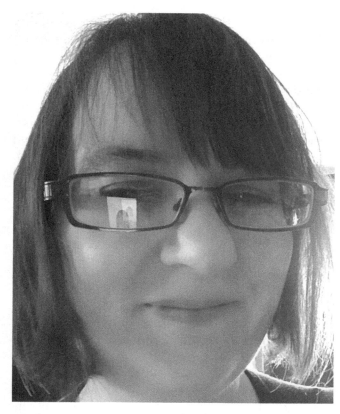

"Still broken and battered, I began once again to care, to believe that I had the power to change this destiny. I decided that I wanted this broken life, and started building a ladder to get out of the pit I found myself in."

There and Back Again - Finding my way out of the dark after diagnosis and disability.

It's so easy looking back, to see the times you could have chosen differently if you'd only known. The times you would have taken the other path had you only known where the one you were walking was headed. The times you should have fought harder, if only you'd known the stakes were so high. The opportunities you'd have seized if you'd realized time to do those things was running out. My unabling came slowly. RA began whittling pieces of my body and my very life away before it was even given a name. By the time I was properly diagnosed, many parts of me were already well on their way to permanent damage.

Within two months of diagnosis, I realized the job I was working at was far too repetitive for my joints to handle. The symptoms were getting worse by the day, as was my ability to keep up with the demands of said job and raising a family. Waking most mornings with hands that refused to open, limping my way through life with an ever-growing list of debilitated body parts, I struggled through each week and then crashed on the weekends, barely able to find the energy to even attempt to keep up with the other demands of life. I knew something had to change. So, I took a leave of absence, promising myself that with rest, targeted exercise, and the treatment plan my rheumatologist and I had made, I would get better and be able to return to work. I believed that until three days before my leave of absence was over. Then reality hit like a ton of bricks. I was not getting better. In fact, I was worse. The medication wasn't working, my hands were hardly functioning, I would not be able to return to the job I'd come to love. The funny thing? Until my supervisor called and asked how I would be able to keep up with my job, I still had been telling myself I somehow could do it. His words were a much-needed reality check. I remember telling him I don't know, and the tears began to fall, as I realized the truth, I was no longer a person who could do that job. So, I resigned, signed the papers later that same week, and then had a good long cry in my car before making the trek home to my new existence.

For a few years, that's what I had, an existence. I was here, but not here. Looking back now, I realize that losing the ability to work sunk me into a rather deep depression. Ability was such a huge part of how I saw myself, to lose it was devastating. I was the kind of person who never thought twice about tackling hard work. The kind of person who often made her own solution with Yankee ingenuity and a little muscle power. And here I was, unable to open a bottle of water. I was lost, I was broken, I was permeated by a deep sadness, and I was SO mad! Mad at the doctors who misdiagnosed me for decades, mad at the medicine that made me feel worse instead of better, mad at the body that had for some reason decided we were enemies, mad at that water bottle I could not open. For years. So, I punished myself. Unable to do whatever I wanted; I chose instead to do nothing I wanted. Frustrated by the things I could not do, I slowly stopped doing everything. Part of me was certain I deserved this, earned it, that it was something I had done to myself. Unfortunately, the internet tended to agree. It promised that if only I took better care of myself, I wouldn't be where I am. Something that alternatively spawned hope and despair in me. Hope for healing, despair for my inability to do enough to make that happen. I was failing my biggest test. I hated myself for it.

Eventually, all that despair and hatred started to show. Rock bottom was approaching. It would arrive shortly after I was approved for disability. Never has a win felt so much like a loss. Never has relief brought with it such deep, dark grief. Disability meant help in the form of income and health insurance, both of which I desperately needed to fight RA. Unfortunately, being swiftly, without any fight, approved for disability, also meant I really was disabled. The words total and permanent leapt off the page. The system had spoken, recovery was no longer expected for me. Reality was devastating.

I soon began to shrink as my depression continued to grow. Before I found my way out of the dark, I would weigh a terrifying 89lbs. A skeletal version of my former self, my outsides now matched my insides, shrunken and hollow. At the time, the weight-loss was a mystery. I had no idea why it had started, even less of a clue how to stop it. The overwhelming hopeless voice that had taken over my psyche was certain I was dying. I will be ever thankful for that thought, whispered in the dark. For finally there was something else blooming in the darkness. Fear. And what does fear do when it awakens in the darkness facing an overwhelming foe? Fear wakes Hope. Needing an ally, it triggers that ever present will to live. Fear rings the alarm and Hope springs into action. Glorious, radiant Hope.

Still broken and battered, I began once again to care, to believe that I had the power to change this destiny. I decided that I wanted this broken life, and started building a ladder to get out of the pit I found myself in. I'd love to say I immediately started gaining weight and feeling better, but that is not how the story goes. It would take many months to begin to see positive changes. At first, I continued to lose. I see now what a blessing that was. How that time allowed Fear to settle in and really give Hope a much-needed kick in the ass. How much I needed to fear losing my life to find the will to fight for it. And find the will I did. Slowly but surely, I began to turn things around. I gained weight, strength, and belief in myself. The stronger I got, the more hope there was. As the number on the scale reached a safe zone, I turned my rediscovered will to fight to other things. I began looking for ways to heal again. I finally remembered who I really was. Glass ½ full, anything is possible, question it all, try anything once, never give up, Tenacious, ME. With hope back at the table, I was able to find the strength to fight for the care I needed, and to begin to put my life back together again.

As I assembled a team of trusted professionals who were truly in my corner, the positive impact of all of those helping hands began to add up. Doing the work led to increased energy and mobility, leaving me free to dip back into the pieces of my life I had ditched on the roadside along the way. I returned to many of the activities I loved, rekindling my long-time love affair with the natural world. As I considered all that I had been through and how much that challenge was due to all that I didn't know, I started toying with the idea of returning to my love of writing as well. Leaning into my science and research background, I started to pull together valuable resources and information for those struggling with a rheumatoid arthritis diagnosis and started sharing my own experience on my blog site. Three years later, I am pleased to have found a way to be able to help others despite the disabilities I battle.

Rebecca Zisk

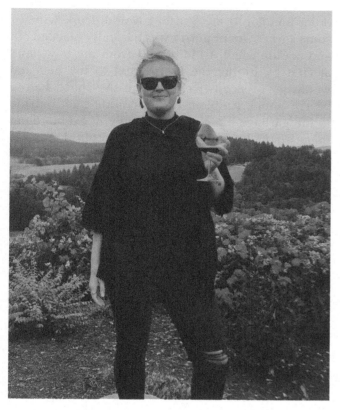

"Life may never be exactly the same as before RA but I have found gratitude. I hope my story can provide hope to someone who is in a position like I once was and give them hope. Please, keep hope alive. DON'T let this disease win."

RA. Where to begin. I was diagnosed in 2019 at the age of 29, two months before my 30th birthday. I spent all of 2018 and the beginning of 2019 working out almost seven days a week and was eating a paleo diet. I had lost close to 50 pounds within that time frame and I was finally in the best shape of my life. I was finally able to wear shorts, cropped tops, and two-piece bathing suits. I had never felt so good physically or mentally. Around March 2019, is when I started to feel physical pain throughout my body, specifically, my feet, knees, wrist, shoulders, and elbows. I would put my feet down on the floor in the morning and I would cry with pain. I could barely lift my arms over my head. My boyfriend Nick and I live together, so he had front row seats to this. I would cry in pain at night just trying to roll over. I couldn't get comfortable, the pain wouldn't stop. I convinced myself that I was just working out incorrectly. Eventually, my boyfriend said he was getting concerned and insisted I make a doctor's appointment. He told me that he hears me crying in my sleep.

My doctor wasn't sure what exactly might be causing the pain so he requested a blood test to be done. 06/29/2019. I was on vacation with my boyfriend in Hilton Head, SC. My phone rings. The results were in.

"I'm almost 100% sure that your pain is caused by rheumatoid arthritis. Your RA factor is a 51."

What? I'm 29 years old? That isn't possible. How? He referred me to a rheumatologist who would make the official diagnosis but he said that he believes this is the cause of my pain. I thought to myself that I could probably take some supplements or get some meds and I'd start to feel better. Oh, how naive I was back then. Little did I know that this was just the beginning of a long fight with this debilitating disease, mentally and physically. Of course, I was put on a 20 mg. dose of good ole prednisone which made me feel amazing. Until it started to make me go crazy and manic. This was temporary until we discussed a medication plan long term. My first RA doctor was awful. His first suggestion was obviously methotrexate, but I said no because the side effects sounded terrible. So I went on hydroxychloroquine with the prednisone, which we tapered down. I felt ok for the first few months. By November, I started to feel pretty awful again but I couldn't get in to see my rheumatologist for months. December was when my left knee swelled to the size of a watermelon. A week or two later, my right knee followed.

By March 2020, the beginning of the pandemic, I was seeking a new Rheumatologist because I found myself wheelchair bound. Unable to walk, unable to shower, unable to lift my arms to get dressed. I cried in agony just trying to lift a cup to drink water. I could barely even grip the cup. My boyfriend had to lift me into bed, brush the knots out of my hair from lying down all day long, physically lift me off the couch and into my chair. Because of Covid, it took months to get in with a new doctor and the combo of meds I was on just did not work (by this point it was orencia and prednisone still). I couldn't even move my hands without my wrists and fingers feeling like they were on fire. If I twisted my wrist my tendons would pop. The apartment my boyfriend and I lived in is 450 square feet, so I could only get to a certain point down the hallway in my wheelchair to use the bathroom. I would have to walk a little bit since the hallway was too narrow. I would use all I had to lift myself, using the walls and whatever I could grab onto, or lean onto, to get me to the toilet where I would have to throw myself down since I couldn't bend my knees. I would sit there way longer than I needed to because I dreaded the thought of trying to stand up. I worked from home, so sometimes I brought my computer to work in the bathroom. We ended up needing to get me a walker to go the extra few steps to the bathroom and to use to lift myself from the toilet. We also got a seat for the shower.

I was 30 by this point and I couldn't even look at myself. I looked nothing like I did in the beginning of 2019. My hair was always a mess, I stunk, I began to gain the weight back. I had a moon face from the prednisone which stopped working at some point. I felt my flare had me too far gone. I spent days awake, unable to sleep from insomnia and pain. Then days where I would sleep for what seemed like forever and I still never felt rested. I thought of how I would get through the next 50 or so years of my life, if I would even live that long with this disease. I started to scream that I was done, I wanted to end it. The things Nick also went through. He went from having an active, fit, happy, funny, goofy girlfriend, to having a girlfriend who was a shell of what she once was. She was angry and severely depressed. He had to bathe me, put me in bed, had to clean the house all by himself, run errands all by himself during a pandemic, and had to worry about getting me sick with Covid while I was just starting a biologic medication.

Our lives flipped upside down. The physical pain I felt was just too much for me. I felt hopeless. No one seemed to be able to help me. My new RA doctor tried what felt like every medication. Every RA cocktail there was. When my boyfriend was able to go back to work after being temporarily laid off due to Covid (he's a chef/bartender), I was left alone at night to take care of myself. That's when the loneliness and depression of this disease really took its toll. Because of Covid, I was able to order alcohol to my house. I would drink wine or some sort of liquor until I was basically blacked out and couldn't feel. I hid it well from my boyfriend at first by hiding the bottle next to my bed and would go to sleep (pass out) on the couch before he got home. Problem was, I couldn't get outside to the garbage bin to throw them out. So he found them when cleaning. After he found out, I stopped caring. I would get so drunk and he would come home and I would scream at him. Telling him he didn't understand, nobody understands. *"Why me!,"* I would scream. I'd scream that I hated my life and that I just didn't want to wake up. I was tired. I couldn't walk, I was in so much pain. It was excruciating. Like fire and razorblades were coursing throughout my body. All my joints were swollen and inflamed. My knees creaked and my left knee started to become knock-kneed. My fingers were starting to turn sideways. Some finger joints were developing nodules.

Life was sad and lonely as a newly disabled person. It was hopeless for a really long time. I am now almost 33 and I'm finally in a somewhat better position thanks to a great team of doctors. I am on methotrexate and enbrel and they keep me moving. Side effects are pretty mild, thankfully. I can walk, which is something I never thought I would do again. I walk with a limp since I did develop severe osteoarthritis in my left knee. I also can't stand for too long without pain. I can't run, which used to be an escape for me. Unfortunately, I am the heaviest I've ever weighed due to being stagnant for so long, but I'm working on it. I'm not 100%, maybe 70%. I am potentially getting knee surgery soon so hope is alive! I have found pleasure in getting to cook again now that my fingers and wrist are functioning. It's become a real hobby of mine. I no longer drink to not feel and my boyfriend no longer has to worry about me when he's at work! He also no longer has to take physical care of me like he once did.

Life may never be exactly the same as before RA but I have found gratitude. I hope my story can provide hope to someone who is in a position like I once was and give them hope. Please, keep hope alive. DON'T let this disease win.

Susan Melanson

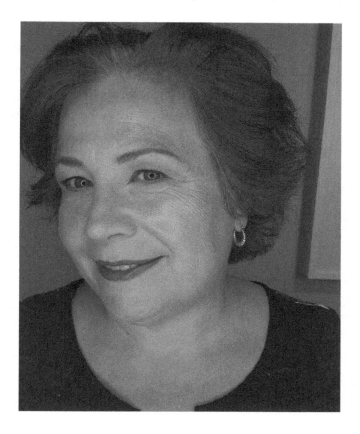

"I consider myself one of the lucky ones."

My Story Starts With A Sore Baby Toe Which I, Of Course, Ignored.

At the time I was newly retired and at the gym five days a week doing spin classes, running, elliptical, and weight training. In the past I had done numerous road races and a couple of Triathlons. I had started agility training with my new dog and was hoping to start competing in that.

After one weight training session I noticed that my knee and shoulder were hurting. I attributed that to poor form because of the sore foot. I decided to see my doctor about the foot. He told me to lose weight and referred me to a podiatrist, and didn't even look at my foot. I couldn't get into the podiatrist for three months, so I found one that didn't require a referral and she took a good look at the foot and sent me for x-rays and an ultrasound. While this was happening my knee and shoulder were getting worse so I found a new GP and she sent me for an x-ray and ultrasound as well.

The results on the knee and shoulder indicated inflammation with no visible cause. We decided to go to athletic therapy for the knee and had cortisone shots for the shoulder, I was also prescribed T3s and NSAIDs. The results for the foot indicated inflammation, so she ordered blood work and gave me a cortisone shot which made a significant impact and I was sure I was cured.

Two months passed and both knees and both shoulders were getting worse. It seemed that the more athletic therapy I did the more painful it got. I was napping several times a day, losing weight at a fantastic rate, pretty much crying all the time and very close to bed ridden.

The blood work came back with no rheumatoid factor but an incredibly high C-reactive protein and white blood cell count. The podiatrist said I need to see my GP right away as something significant is wrong. She mentioned cancer, l, and RA as a few.

I saw my new GP and was sent for more blood work, given a prescription for more T3s and prednisone and they also did an urgent triage to a rheumatologist.

The prednisone seemed to be working as long as the dose was kept high. As soon as I started to taper it I would flare back up to where I was before.

It took five weeks from the time of the rheumatology referral to see my rheumatologist. He went over my history and ordered a ton of blood work, and said I needed a temporal artery biopsy urgently to check for GCA, (giant cell arteritis).

He prescribed methotrexate, folic acid, alendronate, prednisone, zopiclone (sleeping pills). He also recommended I take omega 3s, calcium, vitamin D and baby aspirin. I was given a tapering schedule for the prednisone, as I was only to take it until the methotrexate started working, which can be up to three months. He diagnosed me with RA which I had not considered, as I didn't have a rheumatoid factor. Then I found out about seronegative RA which is what I have.

I had my temporal artery biopsy three days later, and it came back negative, thankfully.

For the next six months every time I got below 20 mg of prednisone I would flare and have to increase it again. My rheumatologist decided to add plaquenil to the mix and remove the baby aspirin. Within three months I was feeling better, and off the prednisone.

I started to eliminate foods from my diet and found that I have less inflammation when I exclude gluten and sugar.

After two years, on this drug regimen and modified diet, I achieved remission and have managed to stay in it for the past two years.

I haven't been able to resume my gym activity. I was spinning and doing some modified weights. I added swimming and hot yoga but both seemed to make my inflammation worse. Then of course Covid hit and, because of my compromised immunities, I have had to limit my outings. I have not been to the gym in two years, although I hope that I will feel safe enough soon to return. I don't think I will be able to achieve my pre-RA level of fitness but that won't stop me from trying.

I consider myself one of the lucky ones, as I have achieved remission and managed to stay in it.

Patricia Blatt

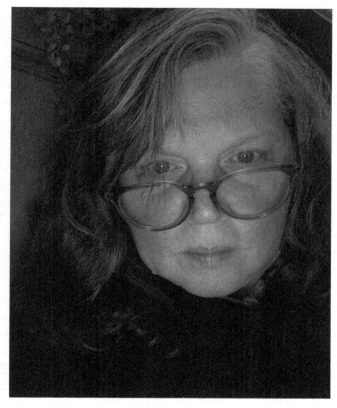

"I conduct my life much like I did before RA, but more deliberately, slowly and with a definite sense of purpose."

I'm a 57 year old mother actively raising four children. My 15 year old son has moderate/severe autism with about 10 other comorbidities. My husband and I adopted three of our grandchildren, ages 13, 11, and 9. My mother with dementia lives with us and my husband was just awarded SSDI, as a result of a back surgery that left his leg numb. I seriously don't have time for my own issues!! But I have to make time, as my GP has said numerous times, "I can't take care of anyone else until I take care of myself."

I was diagnosed with RA in early spring of 2021, and life has not been the same. To be honest, my life has been ever evolving medically, since birth. I have been plagued with autoimmune diseases since infancy, starting with eczema and asthma, and I just keep collecting them over time. I now have seven AI diseases, the last diagnosis of Sjögren's syndrome was about six months ago and it looks like I may also have Raynauds, psoriasis, psoriatic arthritis and lichens sclerosis which round out the AI's, plus ddd. Good times.

I don't feel sorry for myself, I don't have time for that. I move head on to face what is in front of me. Right now, RA is front and center and getting it under control goes a long way in helping to control the other AI's, since many of them are helped by the same treatments. TREATMENT!!! Uggggh, the dreaded scary meds!! Do yourself a favor and don't look up the side effects. It will give you nightmares and convince you that you are going to die trying to alleviate the symptoms that currently occupy your body, and having the disease is better than anything that these drugs could possibly do to relieve your suffering. That just isn't true, and while it is true that there are possible heinous side effects, it is not likely. Any minor side effects will most likely dissipate with time or are not too bothersome. Communication with your rheumatologist is a must, and your Dr will help with side effects or prescribe an alternative. We thankfully live in a time where treatment options are abundant. I am currently on methotrexate and humira. I take 50,000 units of vitamin D3 one time a week, 2,000mg of fish oil for Sjögren's plus xiidra eye drops. I take a muscle relaxer and 75mg diclofenac twice daily. I also take buspirone for anxiety and losartan for palpitations. I also use THC tinctures and full-spectrum CBD for pain and to help with sleep, since during flare it is difficult to sleep. I use Tylenol arthritis for breakthrough flare pain and request prednisone tapers for flares.

Rheumatologist/patient relationships are important. Finding a great rheumatologist is paramount to great care. Unfortunately, it is difficult to get in with ANY rheumatologist as there is a nationwide shortage of specialists, especially rheumatologists. That doesn't mean you have to settle for compassion-less or rudeness. Just know that it usually takes an average of three to six months to be seen. When I prepare to go to my next rheumatology appointment, I keep a log of symptoms on my phone via texts to myself and photos of the swelling in affected joints. I gather them all together the night before so I don't have to fumble for them at the appointment. Lord knows that RA brain fog is real, and I honestly would not remember all the events between appointments if I didn't log them. My rheumatologist really appreciates that I take this step to SHOW my symptoms. Visuals validate what is often very difficult to describe.

Fatigue is my nemesis!! Seriously, f*** my life. I don't have time for the debilitating exhaustion that is inevitable with RA. I was initially diagnosed with MCTD (mixed connective tissues disorder) since I have many crossover symptoms of scleroderma, lupus and RA. It was determined that I definitely have RA, so that is what I am being treated for primarily and as I stated before, the treatment plan for RA helps with the other AI's as well. Along with the cross over symptoms, you guessed it, more fatigue. I have strategies to cope with the fatigue, pain and stiffness that would otherwise throw me into a flare. First of all, I give myself grace. On days when it is all too much, I stay in bed, I don't cook, clean or attend to tasks that can wait. On most other days, I do tasks in 15 minute intervals. It is amazing what can be achieved 15 minutes at a time. I can move mountains, it seems with this strategy. I get the kids involved, they have chores to do and they must do them if they want screen time, friends over, sleep overs or any sort of play time. Since we do chores everyday, it honestly takes them all less than an hour to check off their chores on a chart. It works for us and gives them a sense of responsibility, accountability and pride in contributing to the household's daily operations.

I would say that the most important part of my level of functioning, both physically and mentally, is a good support system. RA is very much affected by stress. We all have stress in our lives coming from numerous sources. Having a good support base by far is the most stress relieving thing in my RA tool box. It saddens me to know that there are so many people who lack support from family, friends and coworkers. I have not worked since December of 2020, due to a hip injury resulting in piriformis syndrome and subsequently an RA diagnosis, but my coworkers, who I have kept in contact with, have been loving and supportive. They have expressed to me how much they miss me and wish I could rejoin our work team. My friends have been great, even though I have to frequently "opt out" of get-togethers due to, not only RA, but my family dynamics. I'm still included and invited even though I most likely won't be joining them. It makes me feel good to know that I am thought of. But...it is a two way street. I am also responsible for holding up my end of the friendship by reaching out, checking in on them too, sending a card or text message letting them know that I am thinking of them "today" and that I am doing my part to keep those connections.

Family support is the most important to me. After all, I live with these people. I seldom complain about my pain or symptoms, they know, they can see it in my face and the way that I have to contort my body just to be able to walk. My 15 year old autistic son is the most compassionate and caring soul and has been the example that the other children follow. He does his chores without being asked and asks me multiple times a day what I need, and what I would like for him to do next. I honestly don't know what I would do without him. My husband is super supportive as much as he can be considering he is disabled. He knows that I am in pain and acknowledges it without trying to one-up me. It's not helpful or necessary when people do this, actually it just pisses people off and pushes them away from you. Of all the things in the world to make a competition about, pain should not be one of them. While I am in some level of pain 24/7, I recognize that there are people who have it much worse than myself. I am grateful that on most days, I can cope. I try not to think too much about the future, one day at a time, or hour or minute at a time is enough to manage. Having a good support system is key in helping me manage all aspects of RA. I am so very grateful for the people in my life and the lift that they give me, I thank them often and specifically for their positive contribution to my life. In contrast, I leave behind toxic people, even if they are family or supposed "friends." I just don't need that in my mental or physical space.

I conduct my life much like I did before RA, But more deliberately, slowly and with a definite sense of purpose. I don't have the energy, time or mental fortitude to waste. There is an old adage in the RA circle about spoons left at the end of the day. You have ten spoons given everyday. How many spoons does it take to do a task? How many spoons to deal with family drama, how many for performing a preferred activity. So we plan, being mindful everyday. When am I going to run out of spoons?

Deb Wilkes

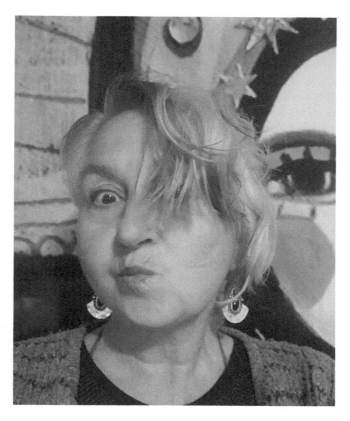

"Guess what? My wrists took the weight of the upper part of my body. I stared in awe. Then tears quietly dripped out of both my eyes."

Humorous Yoga

At 12:30 p.m. on Wednesday morning, I was in Katherine's large garden, half under a gazebo, one eye squinting up to the blue sky watching the clouds lazily move through the gently moving branches of the tree above me, one arm caressing the grass, which was prickly after days of heat.

Last week we worked on abdominals, and I knew I had achieved this as I felt that muscle ache all week. I glowed in the haze of knowing I was using muscles again.

I'd had six weeks of Hydrotherapy with a marvelous therapist, at our local hospital. I'd been told, "You're only 62 and want to dance, kayak and

ride your bike again - let's put you in urgently" she said this to my utter surprise. After weeks of so little activity, I'd seen my arms in a photo and couldn't believe how wasted my muscles had become, I was a withered T-Rex. Katy gave me encouragement that I could regain some muscle, although it may take a while. I left the hot pool feeling positive.

A neighbor suggested, in an energetic and repetitious way, that I join her at "chair yoga." I thanked her but inwardly scoffed at the thought, I either do the hard stuff or not at all. All my life I have felt the need to "be strong" and "pull my socks up," but realized this strategy wasn't working at the moment! After this group there was a small "floor yoga" group, and I guessed I had to start somewhere (whilst also getting her off my case each week!!). All were older than me and had their own creaky bits so I knew there wouldn't be a competition to see who could attain the dizzying heights of the taraksvasana pose each class.

It was midday, so no excuses that I couldn't be ready by then, as I was already beginning to get up earlier – buoyed up on perseverance, anti-inflammatories and the occasional steroid binge!

The stairs there were quite a challenge, then I took my place on a mat, feeling rather exposed and that I wanted to get it over and done with and never go again. In the last few months my exercise regime had constituted trying to turn over in bed (picture quite a bit more than a three point turn, punctuated by small shrieks!) at night and getting to the loo before I wet the bed!

Every RA site was telling me to exercise, when I felt like I actually wondered if I had a form of Tourettes, as every time I moved, my mouth made a noise in protest of my body! Mentally, I was feeling defensive and vulnerable, only good friends and family knew how I had been.

But it was gentle, the music was soothing (and we all started moving yeah, yeah, yeah...) and there was no hint of needing a "perfect pose" (I had sporadically tried other classes over the years). I leant on my forearms, not my wrists (picture awkward) and I knelt on my knees, as my ankles wouldn't hold any weight.

Mainly I moved the bits that I could then crawled up the wall in a valiant attempt to stand upright at the end. My fellow oddbod yogis were quietly encouraging and empathetic, and after a couple of sessions, I let my guard down and allowed myself to enjoy it.

Katherine is a generous character, and lets us sit and have herbals afterwards (teas not the smokes - perhaps I ought to inquire?!) and little bits of personal struggles and triumphs surface, with a group of people I have begun to feel quite close to. They have been alongside me as I have had to work out how to manage my life differently. I have had a weekly dose of stability with them. Next week, we are going to dye each others' hair in different colors.

So back to that Wednesday in the garden...

We were supposed to be doing a downward dog, or something like that pose, and I went to lean on my T.Rex forearms as usual. I looked at my wrists, apart from being brown from the sun they looked the same but I thought I would try them out again. I leaned onto my hands, and tentatively tried to straighten my arms. Guess what? My wrists took the weight of the upper part of my body. I stared in awe.

Then tears quietly dripped out of both my eyes, I almost heard them plop onto the squidgy pale salmon coloured mat. It was like I had come out of my body and was watching, like seeing my baby granddaughter, Noa, smile or roll over for the first time – a magical moment that feels like it will be etched in my memory forever.

Everything stopped for a second and it was as though the last six months of my life flashed by me. The memory of crawling to the bathroom, crying every day because of the shock and overwhelming pain, losing my sense of self, realizing I had a lifelong disease, not wanting to go to bed and not wanting to get up. Then that evaporated and I heard the bids singing.

I dried my eyes with my hand, looked at them all and told them I call this my "Special Needs Yoga for Oldies Group" and it's kept me going. memory

If I couldn't find humor in a situation, I would be a broken woman.

Jenessa Liston

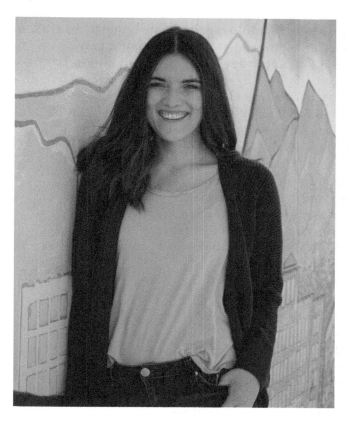

"Losing the body that you thought you'd had is very difficult, but our chronic illnesses can teach us so much and reveal just how strong we really are."

I never cry in public. It feels too intimate, like I'm exposing the core of myself and revealing it to strangers. I reserve that for the unjudging eyes of my shower head, where I can freely release all my fears and doubts through saltwater tears. But today I am breaking this unspoken rule. I have no embarrassment as my rigid body convulses with the force of my sobs. My spine clenches with each sputtered inhale as I struggle simultaneously for breath and release.

I glance up through watery eyes trying to focus on the hospital I just exited. Its behemoth structure rises up, towering over me and mirroring my mood with the dark shadow it's casting. Just two hours prior, I walked through those doors filled with youthful optimism, but despite that hope, I knew something was extremely wrong. I had been experiencing the slow breakdown of my body for several years now. I had sat through countless doctors appointments, watching as their faces crinkled in perplexity while they tried to decipher my labs. I became familiar with the uncertainty edging their voice as they attempted to explain my pain. Sometimes it was dismissed as growing pains, but more frequently, it was delivered through an awkward antidote warning me of the pain associated with texting too much. I left each appointment with the weight of feeling let down. I started to question if I was being too paranoid. But then the pain in my wrists would reach their apex at night, and I would spend countless hours crying from the pain, and vowing that I would keep seeing doctors until they could figure out what was wrong.

As I sat there recovering from my first visit with a rheumatologist, the realization finally sunk in. I had received my long awaited diagnosis. I could finally attach a name to my pain - rheumatoid Arthritis. I whisper it several times letting the name settle on my tongue and sink into my brain. I feel relief that I no longer have to question each new symptom that presents itself. I no longer have to make my own explanations for why I can't grip a pencil, or walk without limping. That relief is immense, but it's also laced with deep sadness. As the name of this disease settles in my brain, the finality of it becomes clear. I can no longer hope for a quick fix. One surgery on my wrist won't completely remove the pain. I know that walking out of those doors changed my life forever. I see a future with medications, pain, and a promise that who I am will change along with this disease for the rest of my life. It's this unknown of who I will become that scares me. So these tears signify the funeral of the body I had before.

I received that diagnosis at the age of 18. I am now 28 years old, and I would love to admit that I only needed to mourn the body I lost for that day, but that would be a lie. I've had multiple breakdowns where my body spasms from the force of my tears escaping my eyes. There is a looming fear at what else is waiting for me in the future. I've already lost the ability to bend both wrists as they slowly fused straight. I've lived through countless days where I've been confined to my bed from relentless fatigue, and I'm awoken several times each night as the eroded joints in my jaw crack painfully.

Grief is an ever present part of this disease, but so is grace. The grace I now have for my body and the strength it continually shows amongst the pain. Grace for other people that have to suffer through the deterioration of their body, whether it's in old age or youth. The grace I've found from other warriors cheering me on through my phone. It's this communal strength of a newfound community that has given me a place of comfort, understanding, and love as we all move forward with this disease. It's this knowledge that I hold onto when the grief comes, that whether or not I'm lying in bed all day, submitting to the rest my body craves, or injecting painful medication into my thigh, I am a warrior for choosing to go through each day with rheumatoid arthritis.

Catalina Ávila Ángel

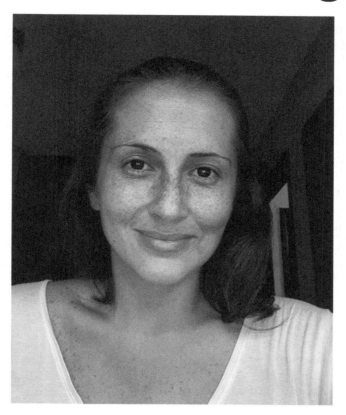

"Finally a diagnosis! My road to discovering a hidden disease and how physical problems turned out to be related to each other."

If only a doctor would have taken the time to relate to my symptoms. If only someone would have figured it out years before. For years I visited many doctors, went through multiple diagnoses, even asked myself if I was crazy or what? Since I was a little kid, I remember having many diseases, and none of them seemed to be related to each other. Something just felt not right, but there was no reason at all. My lymph nodes used to get swollen for no reason, my sublingual gland too. Every time I practiced a sport, something would happen that kept me from continuing. I used to play handball at school,

and suddenly my middle finger started to hurt. It turned out that the tendon was being stuck by a small ball. I had a trigger finger. Then, when I was running, my right foot began to hurt too. Another visit to the doctor, and it turned out, I had a calcaneal spur. After that, I had pain in one knee, and I was also diagnosed with jumper's knee.

By this time, I was 13 or 14 years old and frustration invaded me. How could it be possible that every time I tried to practice a sport, something new would appear? I continued to live my life normally, in pain, without knowing what was going on. Without knowing that what I was feeling was actual pain and fatigue. I just thought I was weak, or I was exaggerating the pain. Migraines, stomach pains, constipation, insomnia. That was me. That's what I felt for years. In my 20's, I was even diagnosed with depression. With psychiatric help, meds, and psychotherapy, I could overcome depression. But again, it seemed like there was no reason for me to be depressed. Years later I got pregnant and had a beautiful daughter. Against all odds, and now that I can consciously look back in time, I actually had a wonderful pregnancy. But even after that, something new was coming. One year before the pandemic, I started feeling pain in one arm. I was laying on my bed, and hadn't done any exercise or anything. It just started to hurt. Again, I wasn't even exercising by that time. I visited a traumatologist. He diagnosed me with golfer's elbow, and saw I had inflammation in my hand. Then the physical therapist diagnosed me with tennis elbow too. I was really frustrated and just asked the traumatologist what was going on with me, why was I having so many physical diseases? He suggested he run some lab tests and x-rays and visit a rheumatologist, just to discard something more serious. But I wasn't ready to know the truth. I didn't want to believe I could have something serious. So, I just ignored what he said and kept going on with my life.

A couple of months later came the pandemic, and my pain was getting worse. I was taking pills every day to relieve my pain. Some days were good, others not so good. And finally, a year after the pandemic started, I decided to visit a rheumatologist, because I began to feel really bad. Not only my arm was hurting. I couldn't even rest when I was in bed. I felt pain every single moment of the day, and the pain was everywhere, in my hands, my arms, my feet, my knees, and more. I wasn't able to sleep either. And then, after a long, long consultation, where I had to specify every single symptom I've had since I can remember, and after seeing my lab tests and x-rays, I was finally diagnosed with psoriatic arthritis.

Thanks to my experienced doctor, who patiently heard every word I had to say, and explained this disease, I was happy and felt good that day. Instead of being in shock, terrified, mad or anything, I was actually relieved. I felt relieved! I wasn't crazy. All the pieces fit in like a puzzle. There was a reason for my pain. Every diagnosis, every symptom, everything had a reason. Now, it's been a little more than a year since my diagnosis. And I must say it's been a hard road. Medications, injections, therapy, ups and downs, flares and good days. I'm finally understanding how my psoriatic arthritis works. And I hope I can overcome every challenge I have from now on. I'm finally accepting that this is a new me. I'm only 32 years old, and I may not be able to do the same things I was able to do a few years before, but I'm getting to know this new me, and now I'm doing things that keep me safe, healthy and happy.

Dana Capsambelis

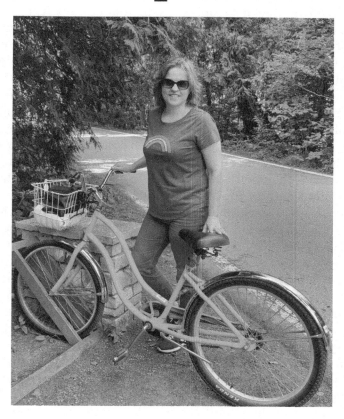

"I have rheumatoid arthritis and osteoarthritis, but it does not define me."

I was diagnosed with juvenile rheumatoid arthritis (JRA) at the age of 12. I had arthroscopic knee surgery at the age of 17. I was diagnosed with osteoarthritis at the age of 20. I had a total hip replacement at age 35. I was in remission (controlled disease activity) for over a decade. I am currently experiencing greater disease activity and am flaring again. I am considering a major medication change. I am a middle aged woman who intends to live a long and glorious life.

When I was first diagnosed as a child, my initial reaction was relief. For some time, I had all of these mysterious aches and pains and swollen joints. I knew something was wrong, and it finally had a name. I remember that my mother cried. She understood the life-long implications of receiving a diagnosis of rheumatoid arthritis. I was unable to comprehend this at my age and inexperience. During my early

years with JRA, I tried many different medications, and I was constantly in physical therapy. I remember that I passed out at school once when I was 16 years old due to a medication reaction. I ran track in high school, and I loved to run. But it took a physical toll on me, and I struggled to keep my joints healthy. Impact sports were hard for me, so my rheumatologist wrote a note for me to take only swim classes and no gym classes. I remember that my physical education teacher thought I was "just trying to get out of gym." I mean, what teenage girl would choose swimming over gym? I never wanted to get my hair wet!

I graduated at the top of my class and went off to college. It was time for me to manage my medications and physical health on my own. College life included a lot of walking. I requested a first floor dorm room to avoid the stairs as much as possible. I continued swimming on campus as physical therapy. It was nice to have easy access to a pool. I developed a great relationship with my rheumatologist and managed my care well as a young adult. Unfortunately, osteoarthritis began creeping in. It was also determined that I now had rheumatoid arthritis (RA), and I did not "outgrow" the JRA.

After college, I married and had three children at the ages of 25, 28 and 30. I worked hard with my rheumatologist to become medication free throughout my childbearing years. I am very proud that I was able to carry and nurse all of my children medication free. Unfortunately, my RA worsened after each pregnancy. Those lovely hormones protected me during the pregnancies, but once they settled back down postpartum the RA would flare. By the age of 32, it was very difficult to walk, and I struggled with constant pain. After seeing hip surgeons, I learned that the years of prednisone use (for my JRA) caused my right hip joint to be destroyed (avascular necrosis). I had no cartilage left. I struggled with the decision to have surgery. I was young, and I knew the recovery would be lengthy and difficult. I put it off for years. These were very painful years as I tried to keep up with my young and active family. I decided at the age of 35 that I could not live with the pain anymore. I found an orthopedic surgeon who would treat me and scheduled surgery. It is difficult to find a surgeon who will agree to do a total hip replacement on a 35 year old, even if she is a very good candidate for such surgery.

Having total hip replacement surgery was the best decision I ever made. Recovery was hard, harder than I expected. But it was all worth it. I felt like I got my life back. I was able to engage in activities again, play with my children, go back to work, take vacations, sleep, and otherwise be present in every way. With time, physical therapy, and medication, I was able to reach a level of remission (symptoms under control). I was stable for eleven years. These were the best years. I always took my medication, but I truly felt a lightness. There was no daily pain and there were no continual worries about the illness. For once, it was not the first thing on my mind each morning and the thing keeping me up at night.

Eleven years after my total hip replacement surgery, I developed tendonitis in my hip (psoas tendon). This is a rare complication of the surgery, and even more uncommon that it appeared so long after my surgery. The daily pain was back, but it was different. There is no cure other than to sever the tendon, which I am not willing to do as it compromises both strength and stability. So, I treat it with physical therapy and rest. This is not a symptom of my RA, but it is a result of my RA.

Unfortunately, I contracted Covid. My illness was more severe than my household members. I attribute this to the fact that RA is an autoimmune disease. Several months after recovering from this illness, my rheumatoid arthritis began flaring again. I was no longer in remission. I am making medication changes to combat these new flares with a hope to again control the disease activity. My rheumatologist felt that my recent flares are directly a result of having the coronavirus. It is very concerning to have fallen out of remission due to this virus, which I tried so very hard to avoid.

At the time that I authored this story, I was a middle aged woman with teenage and young adult children, a loving and supportive husband, a full time career as a social worker, a strong faith, a love of life, and many hobbies. I decided to tell you my arthritis story for multiple reasons. First of all, I knew nothing about rheumatoid arthritis and was provided with very little information about it when I was diagnosed in 1987. The internet did not even exist (imagine that)! I hope that my story helps answer questions about what things might look like in the beginning, and in the years to come. Second, I have felt that it is important to manage my illness throughout my life. I always wanted to understand every option, be a part of the decision making, and invest in the desired outcome. This is your life, do not be afraid to ask questions and share your thoughts and opinions.

Finally, I want you to know that I am Dana. I have rheumatoid arthritis and osteoarthritis, but it does not define me. I am a woman, a mother, a wife, a daughter, a sister, an aunt, a niece, a cousin, a friend, a neighbor, a church member, a social worker, a writer, a coworker, a volunteer, an organizer, a mentor, a collaborator, an adoption advocate, a caretaker, a voter, a patient, a fighter, a homeowner, a business owner, a cook, a cleaner, a shopper, a chauffeur, a party planner, a problem solver, a supporter, a tradition keeper, a candy crusher, a crafter, a reader, a knitter, a baker, a patron of the arts, a porch sitter, a roller coaster rider, a yoga practitioner, a popcorn addict, a chocolate lover, a bicycle rider, a flower smeller, and I AM AN ARTHRITIS WARRIOR.

Liz Contreras Palmer

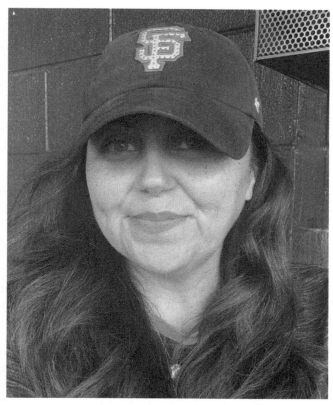

"I run this body, not my disease."

"I Don't Have A Disability. I Have A Different Ability."
—How to run with Arthritis

I t was 2008. I had just been diagnosed with ankylosing spondylitis after six years of experiencing symptoms. I was relieved to put a name to my pain.

Ankylosing spondylitis. Sounds more like a weird dinosaur name than a disease. Oh wait, it is a dinosaur! Ankylosaurus is a dinosaur with an armored back with spikes all over. I guess I found my new spirit animal.

After learning how to pronounce it, I soon got a definition. "It's a type of arthritis that mostly affects the joints in the spine but can cause inflammation in the eyes, hearts, and lungs too."

I thought, so in addition to the back pain and eye pain, I have heart and lung pain to look forward to? But I asked, "What's the cure?" Dr. Diamond responded, "There is no cure yet. We can try medications to slow the disease. But without a cure, you have a 50% chance that your spine will fuse and you will have limited mobility. Honestly, if you can stand it, start exercising, because if you don't move your body, you'll lose it."

It was several years before I decided to become a runner. It seemed to be the only thing I could stick with as a routine exercise, after multiple attempts to go to the gym regularly failed. After I developed a love of running, everything else, diet, cross-training, stretching, and injury prevention, seemed to fall into place too.

But running isn't easy when you are dealing with a chronic disease. So I'm sharing with you the lessons I've learned, that help me to keep moving, while surviving a disease that wants to keep me from doing so.

You do not have a disability. You have a different ability. No, I will NEVER run like a normal person, but I can run. I can still enjoy running even though my body fights this ability. That's because I've decided that I run this body, not my disease. And forward is a pace.

Be mindful of the messages your body is sending you. Some days, I just don't think my body can run. It's not because I don't want to (although that happens too). Maybe I'm just super fatigued (another side effect of this disease) or my back hurts and I don't want to make it worse. Those are the days I take an active rest day instead of running. And I'll postpone my run until my body is up for it.

Tell the negative committee inside your head to shut up and sit down. Sometimes, while running, my mind starts to tell me that I can't run. That I have a disease and I shouldn't be able to do this. That I shouldn't try hard because I'll never be Alyson Felix. That I will never run fast, or run long. So I've learned that these thoughts are wrong and I use them as motivation to keep going.

Motion is lotion. I've decided I'll rest when I'm dead. Until then, I will keep this body moving until there's a cure.

Glenda Monya

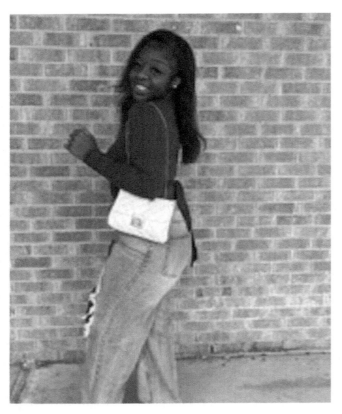

"Arthritis is just a puzzle, you just have to fit it in."

I was diagnosed with arthritis at the age of 14, and since then my life has been one hell of a roller coaster.

It all started on my right hand middle finger, with it being swollen and extremely painful not knowing what happened. From there it just started spreading with pain throughout my body everywhere. I didn't understand what was happening to my body at that age. I just thought it was growing pains and it'll pass but it was not growing pains at all, far from it. It was a lot to process especially at that young age as I just didn't know what was going on with me and the sucky part about it, is that it only got worse before it got better.

It was just like a really bad roller coaster, it just kept going down. I felt like my body was not my body. It was like an endless uncontrollable drop. I felt weak, tired, and stiff all of the time and it sucked so bad.

Without my diagnosis I was constantly suffering as I was not my normal self at all, my energy, motivation, and mind, just not me. My family noticed it and they knew as well. It was a lot and I was suffering. It was after my diagnosis where things started to get better, but it was still rough.

My arthritis started in my wrists and elbows and it has now settled in my left knee and hips. The pain is never the same and it changes constantly day by day. I've been managing my pain with different medications. I started off with methotrexate, enbrel, prednisone, and naproxen, that combination alone was a lot on my body, especially my mind, as I was still trying to understand why I have to take all of this to feel some type of better. With time it did get better, but that roller coaster was still going downhill as I did not know exactly what I was going to face later on.

The healthcare system is the greatest on kids with preexisting conditions and I am one that is facing that problem. There were times I wasn't able to get my medication, just simply because something with my insurance went wrong and they wouldn't cover it. With that it started to turn into the spiral of me going back to where I started in the beginning and that honestly just sucked. I ended up getting off of all four of those medications and started taking humira and 800mg Ibuprofen. It has been working with me, but no medication is perfect. Also with time it started to settle more in my hips and that started a new set of problems for me.

In 2020, I ended up having a total hip replacement with my right hip. Although I was happy some of the pain was going to be relieved, it was still a lot to process and go through. I recovered quickly, but I still don't like feeling helpless or being in pain. It is just always how I am.

Today I am doing so much better, but like any kid with arthritis the obstacles and challenges are endless. With it all I just start to see them as puzzles and just trying to fix the pieces in the right spot. I'm just taking it step by step and piece by piece. I wouldn't say this illness hasn't stopped me from doing things because it has. I can't sit criss crossed anymore, jump, run long distances, and so much more. Although I can't do these any more I don't dwell on it and I just find new things to do.

With time I've accepted it is a part of my life and I can not really do much about it, other than just make it fit into what my life already is now. It's a puzzle really, it's all a process of just seeing where it fits.

Estelle Gleave

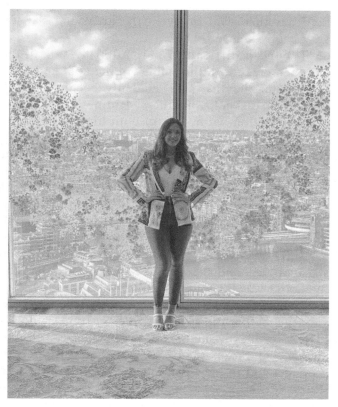

"When I had my first flare up in January 2021, it soon became clear that paracetamol and ibuprofen were not going to cut it, the changes I/we had to make were rapid."

It took just over eleven months to reach a diagnosis in the early post- pandemic UK, with an exhausted and overwhelmed National Health System (NHS), and an economy heading towards the brink of collapse.

When you say it out loud, eleven months doesn't seem like a long time, but it felt like an eternity with my main concern being, that at some stage, I was going to get a phone call to tell me they had detected something more sinister, as I could not imagine being debilitated by so much pain could ever be called by arthritis.

Surely that's something for old people caused by repetitive strain over the years- right?... Please tell me I'm right.

Wrong.

Following my diagnosis, the changes I had to make in my life were rapid because of the overwhelming impact the disease had already had on simple things I had taken for granted.

There's certainly things in my house that make sense now that I'm an RA gal. Cushioned vinyl floors, electric blankets, my bargain recliner chair... and I wish the changes stopped there.

However, in reality rheumatoid arthritis has threatened to shake the core of all the things that I have worked hard for and hold dearest to me.

Primarily, my own little family that had just begun to grow after so much hope and heartache. This is perhaps the hardest change of all. And it tugs on my heartstrings daily.

I can remember in the early days when my hubby, being the grafter that he is, had gone to work before anyone else was awake. I woke up one morning to my one year old son calling me from his room to tell me it was time to get up. Normally, I'd have thought nothing about stepping out of bed, fetching my dressing gown from the back of the bedroom door and carrying him downstairs. But this morning wasn't a regular morning, and I found myself stuck in bed, barely able to lift my head off the pillow, shouting, *"Morning! Mummy's on her way!"* In reality I was thinking how am I ever going to make it to my son.

My husband made sure to be around in the mornings to help and also did the majority of the carrying him to bed, on top of all the other heavy parenting. On occasions when he was away, my mum flew in from Ireland to be on hand to help, which wasn't ideal in the middle of two lockdowns and constant travel restrictions.

I used to get so upset thinking I'd never have the chance to carry him to bed again. Even worse, by the time I got well enough he'd be too old to want to be carried up to bed. But luckily, 12 months on I've had plenty of opportunity, even if sometimes climbing the stairs is not the smoothest of transactions!

It's certainly made the motherhood experience a lot more lonely. There are lots of parks and soft plays that are no go zones for me on the days I have off with my son. I worry that if he had a good old tots tantrum, that we'd physically never make it back to the car, or if he went too fast, too high or got stuck, I wouldn't be able to get to him in time before, heaven forbid, there was an accident.

Luckily, I have worked out a good list of go to's that we enjoy. And we visit the others as a family when we're all together so we never miss out.

As well as my family, RA has also reared its head and has woven its way into my career. I began teaching in 2011 and am responsible for PE and sport at my school which I teach in several classes.

My work has been amazing at supporting me through this journey and have brought about several changes that help. They were the first to see me become ill right at the beginning of lockdown 3.0 and always looked out for me.

They saw how frustrating it was trying to reach a diagnosis and reached out to Occupational Health (OH) on my behalf, to see if there was anything they could do to help in the meantime. This helped them to put together a risk assessment that included thinking about safe storage of medication and painkillers whilst in work, which I hadn't considered at the time.

They even let me choose my own special chair which was fun at the time. OH recommended an ergonomic saddle chair with a back support (Google it, it's hilarious), to which I replied not a chance! It was bad enough hobbling around in front of my colleagues, without wheeling around on something that wouldn't look out of place in a museum in Amsterdam.

Now I have a slick chair that helps when working at different levels and has made a difference to knee and hip pain at work. It helps to be comfortable but I do feel that embarrassment and shame creeps in the most in work, which is a place where I like to feel respected and equal to the people I in turn respect around me.

I always try to arrange my appointments for days when I'm not at work but with certain clinics that's not always possible. Attending appointments has never been an issue, even when I felt like I was inconveniencing my colleagues. When another letter comes through for another Thursday morning appointment, I can't help but feel the dread that I need to make another dash out of work, even though they've made this as easy as possible for me.

In between working and being a mum, the other biggest responsibility in my day to day life is my horse. My dream has always been to have my own horse and I've been lucky enough, not only to

achieve my goal, but to have a mare I've loved for a long time. My friends allowed me to bring her over in 2013 and she's been with us since. When I first became ill, we were on a DIY contract at a yard with facilities that rival many in the area, and she was very happy and settled.

I found it difficult to look after my son all day and then make it to the stables in the cold and damp late winter months, so I suddenly became heavily reliant on the help of others. Riding was also out of the question, with pain in both hips, both knees, bursitis in both ankles, swollen fingers and not being able to turn my neck due to crippling shoulder pain.

My husband is well versed in mucking in to muck out, so he would go after being at work all day. My amazing friend would help out several days a week and took over the riding. I also had the help of several liveries I'd become close with and could use staff services as well, but I always had a niggling sense of guilt and shame that I couldn't give back all the help I was borrowing.

I made the decision to move to an assisted livery yard just before the second winter of living with RA kicked in. It is a smaller, beautiful family run yard and one of the major perks was that it offered all year turn out in the fields, which meant that had my illness struck as bad as it had the previous winter, she could still get out and have time to roam.

It was a tough decision as it meant taking her away from my friend, who had been so good to us, and a yard that she had spent four happy years at. But thankfully, she settled really well and I couldn't ask for better care for her during the week. My friend has also popped round to visit!

The yard is close to miles of bridle paths which allows me to still keep in touch with riding, without having to solely rely on schooling in an arena, which can be heavy going on the joints in my legs.

So far, the changes have been manageable and luckily I've had an abundance of help and support from the people around me. Although I feel with each compromise there is an undercurrent of guilt, embarrassment or worry that I'm not able to be fully the person I once was.

I find it so tough to ask for help and worry that people think I am lazy, but I think that's on me. I'm still finding ways around living with an invisible illness but I realize how much others have been here for me, and that me and my life are so much more than arthritis.

Johana Medina

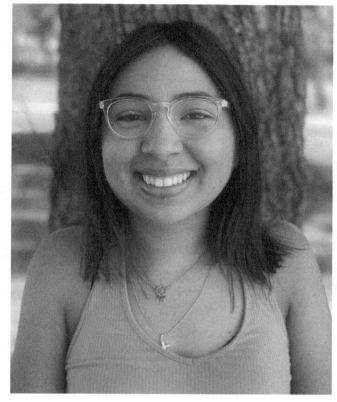

"Never, Never, NEVER give up on yourself...like ever!"

I had my first ever flare when I was eighteen years old in 2018. I was still in high school and had just gotten out of my weight training class. And by the time I walked to my next class, my wrist was swollen. The next day my knees and lower back started to hurt as well. I really didn't think much of it except for, "oh man I must have injured myself in weight training class, I'm gonna have to rest for two weeks." (I wish it was two weeks right!!). But little did I know that I would be searching for a diagnosis for more than three years after that day. I experienced medical gaslighting for years until I was finally diagnosed at the end of 2021.

After some pains, I went to my primary care doctor at the time, who said it was a "sprain" and sent me to physical therapy for a few months. When that didn't help I went back and persisted for something else, an MRI, blood test... anything!! I was sent back to physical therapy, meanwhile my day to day activities were getting more difficult to accomplish. Writing my notes for school was absolute torture. I tried to get some accommodations at school, but without a medical diagnosis they refused to give me any help. When I asked to be transferred to another dr, I asked her if I could be referred to a rheumatologist? In March of 2019 (during the time when Covid was crazy!!) I finally got to see a rheumatologist. She ordered x-rays and blood tests, but two weeks later she called me and said, "that at this time" she does not believe I have any sort of autoimmune disease. Perhaps my joints are just a bit "flexible."

I felt shattered and hopeless; I knew something was wrong with me, but I couldn't get any dr to take me seriously. As time went by the pain got so bad I couldn't even walk a couple of steps. Week after week I would experience more and more pain and new symptoms. When I went back to my primary care doctor, desperate for answers, she told me that she would "advise me to go on an antidepressant for a while." I was put on two different antidepressants. I refused to give up and saw orthopedic, genetics, more physical therapy etc. All of the doctors told me I'll be ok, "you're healthy," you're very young for the pain you're describing."

During this time, I never felt so alone in my life. I would think about ending my life everyday. I just wished someone would believe me. In my last hope I went back to the rheumatologist. She once again did more blood tests and an MRI of my back, which had now had a lot more damage. Two weeks later I was diagnosed with ankylosing spondylitis. Medical gaslighting had and still has a huge impact on my mental health. My doctors not taking me seriously put me in a position where I felt hopeless, because I had no idea what was going on with me.

I still go to therapy to cope with my diagnosis and the gaslighting that I experienced for over three years of my life. Since receiving my diagnosis, I have learned how to advocate for myself and always do what is best for me. I always know now when I am being medically gaslighted and always advocate for myself when it occurs. Looking back on those years of my life, where I didn't know what was going on, I feel very angry and sad. But I'm also very glad I never gave up on myself when it felt like everyone did. It has also taught me to always, always put myself first because no one else will.

Stephanie Sloan

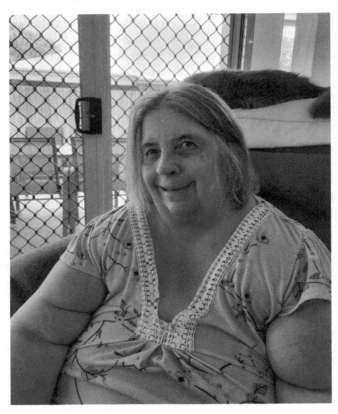

"Take one day at a time."

My primary diagnoses are severe rheumatoid arthritis and psoriatic arthritis. I also have osteoporosis and osteoarthritis. It took my doctor from 2001 to 2016 to fully diagnose my RA. I am in my 50's and I am married with three sons. My PSA was diagnosed in 2020.

I was on methotrexate and simponi but my body didn't like the simponi injection. I had every side effect and it caused severe ulcers. I have had 11 orthopedic surgeries. My foot surgery failed the first time and I had cellulitis infections. They did a second operation on my foot which was successful but I still had infections.

I use a walker around the home or for short distances. I use a power wheelchair over a long distance. My hubby also has a wheelchair which is faster than mine. We both have a National Disability Insurance Plan (NDIS), which is an Australian Government financial assistance package, providing care for people with severe disabilities. We also have a great physiotherapist.

Due to the severity of my disease, we live in Specialist Disability Accommodation, which is housing provided as part of our NDIS plan. It has overhead hoists and full wheelchair access. The house is solar powered and the doors and blinds are electric. I have professional carers to look after me.

I have chronic pain. My pain flares once or twice a month, often because of the change in weather. Sometimes I feel stressed and anxious. I have brain fog and extreme fatigue. Also, sometimes I wake up and get out of bed but I can't get in by myself.

(This story is dedicated to Stephanie's husband, who sadly passed away on the 19th of August 2022).

Emilia Leonetti

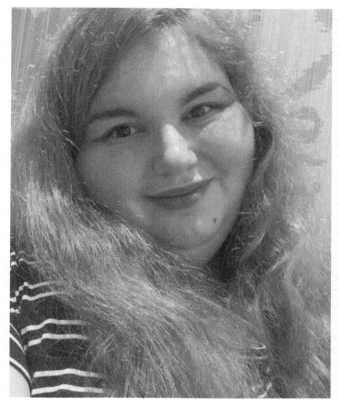

"A wheelchair to help with my mobility would be a dream come true, but I still don't feel "disabled enough" to own one."

I still remember exactly when I had my first flare-up.

While living in hilly Tasmania with my family, I used to take our dogs out for walks. The little walking trails branching off from our street were our favorite – a creek snaked beside us as we trekked between trees and over wooden bridges.

One day, I felt a sharp pain in my lower back and immediately had to sit down on a nearby bench. The resulting discomfort was almost unbearable – but with effort, I was able to walk us all home.

At the time, I was 24 years old. As of writing, I'm 28. In the intervening years, the pain only got worse. I brushed it off with youthful arrogance, thinking extra exercise would somehow cure me, but it didn't. When I was living in a Sydney share house in 2019, I found it difficult to even walk to the bus stop on the main street, about 800 meters away.

Just recently, I was diagnosed with osteoarthritis in my lower back. I've had knee problems since I was 12, but I still found it relatively easy to walk, albeit with a limp. However, it wasn't until recently that the pain spread to my lumbar region. Although I'm glad to have the terminology to describe how and why I've been in pain for a long time, I can't shake this loss. When people see me, they see a bigger person – but in spite of the stereotypes about us, I used to love walking long distances. Now I struggle to walk to the end of my street without feeling a burning desire to sit down. Because of how recent my diagnosis was, I am only just beginning my journey of looking into treatment options, and I'm desperately hoping for something that can effectively treat my pain.

I'm still active, but every workout I do has to be seated with limited standing options. I've been focusing a lot on my core strength, by doing Pilates and other such exercises, to manage my pain and strengthen my body so I don't end up atrophying.. I'm trying to take care of my physical and mental health as much as I can in the hopes that my efforts will pay off.

One day when I was at the airport, I had a flare-up while going from one gate to another – airlines can be annoying with their last-minute gate changes. Seeing my desperation, some of the airport staff got me a wheelchair. It was a game-changer. I felt so comfortable, I almost cried tears of joy.

A wheelchair to help with my mobility would be a dream come true, but I still don't feel "disabled enough" to own one. However, I'm trying to unlearn my internalized ableism in this regard. Osteoarthritis is a degenerative disease and I'm fully aware that it won't get better anytime soon. One day I'll be able to manage my pain effectively, and I live in hope that I can still live a full, joyful life with the disability I've acquired.

Linda Olbort

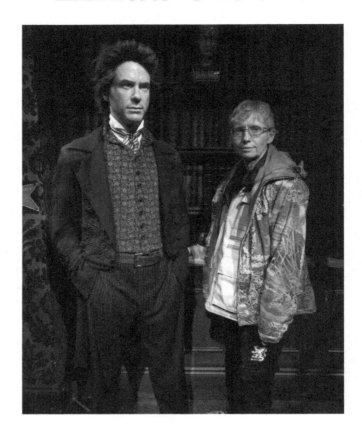

"Roller coaster ride of pain, disabilities and multiple surgeries. But I am still standing!"

It was a hot summer day when at age six, I dove into a swimming pool and hit the bottom, snapping both wrists back, but not injuring them. Six months later began a roller coaster ride of pain, disability and multiple surgeries. 64 years of RA suffering, doing activities I love, losing them and finding new activities to love.

Physiotherapists became my new best friends as they guided me, helped me to do whatever it took to keep moving and not lose ground against the disease. I credit them for keeping me out of a wheelchair, when at age 24, I had a massive full body flare in every joint and was bed ridden. Six months in the hospital with daily, intensive physiotherapy got me from barely being able to walk or move to going two blocks. I love physical activity and always got back into it when the flares ended. When I couldn't do martial arts as a teen, I took up gym classes. I hiked and then enjoyed paintball. When I could no longer play paintball, I enjoyed step, boxercise and Zumba workouts. I have had seven joint replacements, one failed after only three years, but I maintain my weight and an active lifestyle. I have had some 48 surgeries and every joint in my body has been damaged by RA and osteoporosis. But I am still standing.

Allison Buchanan

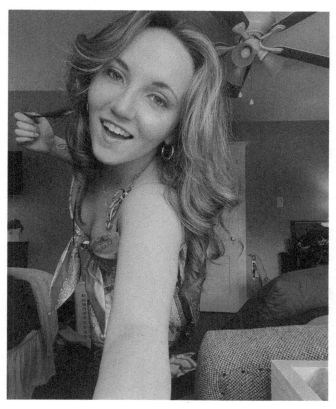

"I want people to understand that arthritis affects people of all ages and it's more than just joint pain."

My mother and my brother both suffer from psoriatic arthritis, and unfortunately, they passed it down to me. I was diagnosed when I was 17 years old, but it took 10 years of misdiagnoses and a LOT of, "you're too young for arthritis," to finally get there. Living with joint pain and swollen knees is something I've grown used to, but no one realizes the other dangers that come with having arthritis, such as the risks we take by going on biologics to control our autoimmune disease. In 2019, I was being treated with enbrel until one week I became sicker than I've ever been before. I was rushed to the hospital with a 105 fever, a rash all over my body and my vitals nowhere near normal. The night before I went into the hospital, I dreamed that I was fighting for my life because that's what it truly felt like. After maybe 50 tests and seeing multiple doctors, I was diagnosed with toxic shock syndrome due to my weakened immune deficiency from the enbrel. I didn't even know it was possible to get TSS without a tampon. Being treated for that was one of the scariest things I've ever gone through and today, my doctors and I still struggle to find the right treatment for me and my body. I am about to start cosentyx this week, which will be the third treatment I've been on since the enbrel.

As a young adult living with arthritis, no one truly understands what you go through every day, except myself and my rheumatologist. My mother and brother also suffer from psoriatic arthritis which is very nice to have other people around you who know exactly what you're going through. I'm also extremely thankful for my incredible rheumatologist who continues to find a way to ease my pain every day. I want people to understand that arthritis affects people of all ages and it's more than just joint pain. I also want to share my story for all the young people out there living with arthritis. I want them to know that they are not alone as that is something I wish I could hear more often.

Jennifer Weaver

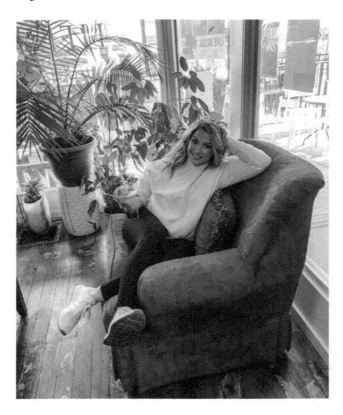

"We can do hard things!"

My first Rheumatologist began treating me with disease modifying drugs as he believed I had an autoimmune disease of some kind. I had several reactions with the worst causing a seizure. Ultimately, I switched rheumatologists after no diagnosis and my treatments had gone so wrong.

The new team quickly diagnosed me with RA. We found a combo of methotrexate and actemra to try. My body was not tolerating it as in some cases it may cause you to have a lower number of certain white blood cells that help fight infection. After much debate we tried remicade. Talk about treatments gone wrong! Exposure to certain drugs can elicit an induction of pustular psoriasis. I have an allergy to TNF Inhibitors that we were unaware of. I share my story to help others know they are not alone and that you can still live a semi-normal healthy life, with a great care team and treatments.

Katie Kumpulainen

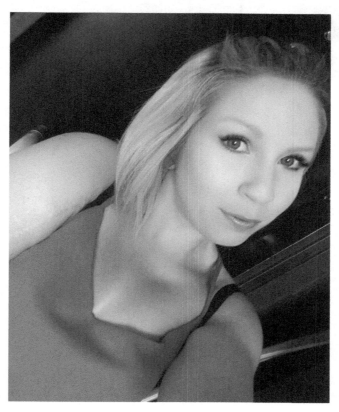

"Healing is possible, please keep your heart and mind open. If medications don't work, try another way."

I want to tell my story of my healing journey. I had big losses in the autumn of 2018. My dog died, I lost my best friend, I changed jobs. The job was everything else than a dream job when it started. Super stressful environment. Work buddies bullying me, the CEO was a narcissist, etc.

I got my RA diagnosis in the summer of 2019. I also got my fibromyalgia diagnosis after that in August 2020. I had different pains all over my body and I was not able to move. Electric shock pains, nerve pains, RA pain for example. Pain every day, they were hard days. We tried many RA medicines in these years, and everytime I got bad side effects. Same thing happened with fibromyalgia medications. I was in a wheelchair for a little bit over one and a half years. I got different hand and neck supports. I was not able to cook, wash my hair, walk, I couldn't do anything. Just be at home.

I stopped all medication in September 2021 because they just made me moon faced, my body was like a balloon and they didn't help me. They just gave me a negative shape image, more pains and illness.

I heard about Medical Medium for the first time in 2019. Wow, just with food, mental balance and balancing your life from stress, you can heal? Yeah right. So I started to remember what kind of food I ate and the stress in my life etc. I started with baby steps to eat more healthily and ignore and remove all negatives from my life.

Now in 2022 I can say to you this protocol saved me and I am pain free. Last autumn I played badminton like I used to in 2018. Healing is possible when you know the root cause for your illness. Processed food, dairy, eggs, wheat, msg, stress etc, are the worst for our health. I am healing, I know you can heal too!

WORK, CAREER & FINANCE

Stories

Georgie Wishart

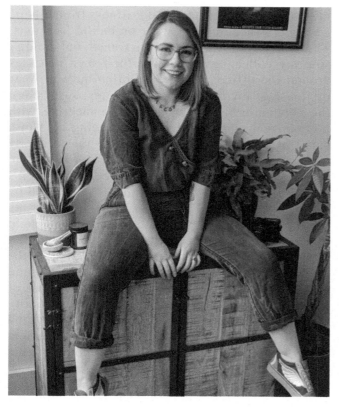

"Before my arthritis diagnosis, and even for a few years afterwards, I would have seen reducing my hours and my 'productivity' as a failure. But success looks a little different to me now."

The Glass Ceiling

I am a textbook overachiever. A stereotypical, ambitious Capricorn. I have always measured my worth by how well I did in school, what jobs or promotions I've secured, how high my salary is... But I never felt satisfied with any of it.

As a woman of the Y2K generation, I no longer had to focus on bagging a desirable husband and becoming a housewife. I was taught I could achieve anything that I wanted. We were actively encouraged to break the glass ceiling (as long as you didn't mind being paid less than your male counterparts). And that's what success meant to me - being a #GirlBoss.

So when I was diagnosed with inflammatory arthritis at 28, you can imagine how I reacted. This was just another challenge that I would have to overcome. "Finally we can make a plan and I can crack on with my goals," I thought, after six long years of undiagnosed pain and mobility struggles. Unfortunately for me, degenerative chronic illnesses aren't fixed that easily. And despite giving my arthritis both barrels of medication, and lifestyle changes, this condition impacts every aspect of my life.

My first symptoms were pain and muscle spasms in my lower back. They appeared sporadically and so I was usually given NHS physio and hoped it would be fixed this time - but over the next half decade, my undiscovered condition really began to take its toll. My partner often had to lift me out of bed in the morning, and help me put on my underwear because I couldn't bend down without screaming. I would have to take over the counter opioid painkillers so that I could make it up the stairs at my local train station in the morning. I may have been in my late twenties, but I often felt like a frail eighty year old. It became so overwhelming that I finally had to acknowledge that I couldn't carry on like this. I couldn't just keep plowing on as though I was fine. I wasn't fine.

As you can imagine, it was also having a huge impact on my work. My primary inflammation lies in my SI joints, so sitting at a desk for eight hours a day was challenging for me. I bought a coccyx cushion for my chair, a plug-in heat mat, and I kept a variety of ointments and pills in my desk drawer - all of which helped a little. Then my disease began to spread outwards to my hands, my feet, my knees, and my elbows. So I added compression gloves for typing, support socks for my ankles, and physio tape to give my joints extra support on bad days. I'd stand up during meetings as I couldn't sit for long periods. When my colleagues asked if I was okay, I'd just say that my back hurt. You might be wondering why I didn't ask for support from the Human Resources department. How could I when I couldn't give any explanation for why these things were happening to me? Plus our Head of HR was generally apathetic... and borderline malodorous.

Eventually, after years of hassling my GP, I was referred to rheumatology at the local hospital who ran a number of tests, and they diagnosed me with spondyloarthropathy. Finally having a diagnosis helped me feel more in control and I now had strong evidence to back me up if I needed to ask for any support at work. I even downloaded the National Axial Spondyloarthritis Guide For Employers, and emailed it to my manager and the HR department, alongside my new diagnosis, so they could learn more about my condition.

There was a strict sickness policy at that office - we were only allowed to take a small number of sick days per year before disciplinary action was taken. We also weren't permitted to work from home, which meant that even on my worst days I would have to drag myself across North London, on top of a full day in the office. I would also regularly sit at my desk during a flare, a fever raging through my body, and I would feel so unwell that I'd have to lie down on the grubby meeting room floor until the worst of it passed. My team was incredibly understanding, but why was I put in that position in the first place?

Anyone who struggles with their joints will know how strongly they are affected by temperature. That particular office was freezing in the winter and scorching in the summer. In fact, one time it reached 38 degrees celsius, so I requested to work from home for the rest of the day where I could stay cool. Preferably answering emails in my pants with an endless supply of ice lollies. But I was met with a firm no. That evening, my friend with Crohn's disease was physically sick, and I ended up at the doctor with heatstroke. In the colder months, my joints would seize up and become a lot more painful, so I purchased my own portable radiator, which I put next to my desk. On its discovery, I was given a stern talking to. And in spite of explaining about my pain and stiffness I was experiencing, I was explicitly told it was not to be plugged in. Reader, I plugged it in every day.

But the most difficult challenge for me came when I started taking biologic therapy to treat my arthritis. I was extremely hopeful that this treatment would stop the progression of my disease and decrease my inflammation. But the downside was that it would leave me immunosuppressed and susceptible to infection. My office, like many others, had a culture of presenteeism, so most people would come into work when ill. So when I started my biologic injections, I sent a vulnerable email to my office explaining my situation and that I would appreciate a quiet heads up if someone was unwell, so that I could keep my distance. I often wondered if anyone had actually received the email because my request was ignored.

So it was unsurprising that I caught a cold from someone in my office soon after I had started the medication. It quickly turned into bronchitis, which had to be treated with steroids. To reduce my risk of catching even 'mild' illness from others, I bought a face mask to wear on public transport. This was helpful whilst I was in transit, but it didn't stop my colleagues spreading their own illnesses around the office. So I would often have to wear my mask at my desk and in meetings. Just before the pandemic began, I went into a meeting with my manager and the CEO. It was being held in a small office so I chose to wear my mask, as my manager had a streaming cold. When we sat down, she looked at me, laughed in my face and said "It's not that serious." It wasn't for her, but it could be for me.

It became clear that I wasn't going to be able to manage my condition, the way I wanted to, whilst in traditional employment. The bureaucracy, the presenteeism, the lack of understanding around disability and chronic health conditions... all of these things stood between me and a better quality of life. So in the winter of 2019, I decided that I needed to take more control of the management of my condition, and I handed in my notice with a heavy sigh of relief.

The best part is - I still get to do the job I love. I started a freelance business where I provide the same marketing and communications services, but for lots of different, amazing charities. What's more, I run my business the way I want and I am able to put my health first, even when the overachiever in me finds that difficult. If I need to have an Epsom salt bath or have a nap in the middle of the day, I will. I don't have to waste hours of my life commuting. I'm even able to work shorter hours and still get the same amount of work done, because I'm not dragging it out to fill the 9-5.

Before my arthritis diagnosis, and even for a few years afterwards, I would have seen reducing my hours and my 'productivity' as a failure. But success looks a little different to me now. I'm not measuring my worth by the amount of tasks I get done or the amount of money I make. It's putting myself and my health first. It's enjoying a quiet cup of coffee in the morning with my dog, or waking up without swollen joints. I may not have broken the corporate glass ceiling, but I have broken through my old mindset and into a better way of life.

Stefanie Remson

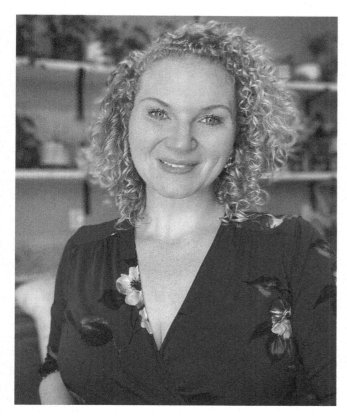

"Don't be afraid to pivot!"

I'm a happily married mother of two young boys. I'm a nurse practitioner (NP) with over 15+ years of experience. I have rheumatoid arthritis (RA).

Before you sigh with sadness or anticipate the weight of my sob story, hold on for this incredible ride! I'm about to share a very unexpected tale about my life after my RA diagnosis.

I was diagnosed with RA when my first son was just a few weeks old. I struggled to feed and care for him after he was born. The pain in my hands and wrists was crippling. At one point I lost function of my left hand almost completely. I called it my "barbie hand" because it was so stiff and useless! Holding a bottle, or changing a diaper, was impossible. I was constantly asking the people around me for help.

After my maternity leave, I returned to my job as a NP in a large hospital with very critically ill patients. The job was physically demanding with long walking distances, stairs, heavy lifting, standing for long periods, and lots of procedures with tiny, sterile instruments. I dedicated my life to helping others when I became a nurse practitioner, and I wanted to do only good. I was so torn when my body could not meet the physical demands of the job anymore. I had so many emotions: anger, denial, grief, sadness, anxiety, frustration. No matter how I looked at it, or what I felt, I simply could not keep up.

I was a young person with this amazing career in healthcare that I had worked so hard for. So many years of schooling, travel, testing, etc. I had made so many sacrifices to get there. I felt like it was shattered right in front of my eyes. I was afraid... No... I was terrified! I was afraid for my professional future, my son's future, and my ability to generate income. I became depressed and fell into a state of hopelessness and despair. I was in a really dark place.

One day I was especially panicked and unsettled about my unpredictable professional future. I ran into a professional mentor of mine. In private, I disclosed to her that I was recently diagnosed with RA and my physical limitations were too great to continue in my current role. In a short and sweet sentence she said, *"You'll be fine— you'll have a new job tomorrow!"* She motioned vaguely all around her as though to say there's a new opportunity on every corner! And that was that... she ended the conversation. I went home, applied for a variety of other NP positions and waited. I got a call back almost immediately from three places I had applied. I gave notice, left on good terms, and completely changed directions in my career. I call this my big pivot.

I accepted a position in a primary care office. They made me an incredible offer that I couldn't refuse. The health benefits were amazing and the schedule was much more flexible for my growing family. I still couldn't believe that this forced pivot could lead to great things. I spent the next five years excelling in this NP position.

When the Covid pandemic hit, I received a call from an old friend who is an infectious disease physician. Believe it or not, I made another huge pivot! I left primary care to go work in infectious disease, during a global pandemic! It was the craziest thing I have ever done, but oh so rewarding! The courage and strength came to me unsolicited! At the time, there wasn't a doubt in my mind. I knew that I could handle the challenge. I also knew it was the right move for me. Right place, right time! I don't think I would have had the confidence to do something like this if it weren't for my diagnosis of RA so many years ago. In a way, RA has shaped me for the better. RA made me stronger, more resilient, and more adaptable to change.

When I was diagnosed, I felt very lost and alone. I couldn't believe the lack of resources and support there were for people with RA, and I was a medical professional! This was my life's work. This was what I had devoted my life to. At the same time as my big pivot, I also started volunteering with the Arthritis Foundation. I led a very successful, and popular, support group for people with arthritis. Many of them had RA, just like me. It was an incredible experience that allowed me to connect with others for my own needs, but also to offer support to others with chronic pain and RA. It was so rewarding to give back to the arthritis community. I met amazing people through this group and many have remained life-long friends. I never would have met them if it were not for my diagnosis, my job change, and my new schedule which allowed me the luxury of time to volunteer.

Would you believe me if I told you there was more good that came to my professional life, because of my RA diagnosis? It's hard to believe, but here it goes!

Shortly after my big pivot and the birth of my second son, I founded Rheumatoid Arthritis Coach. At Rheumatoid Arthritis Coach, we work with people one-on-one to better manage their symptoms of RA. We get people back to living again! I have made the biggest career pivot ever! Now I help people live fulfilling, gratifying lives despite RA! What a gift! I am so honored and humbled to serve this community each and everyday. I never could have done it without my diagnosis of RA.

Although the diagnosis of RA was devastating at the time, so much good came from my big pivot! I made the best of a tough situation. I am so proud of how far I have come professionally. I had no idea RA was going to make me this much stronger!

I made a big professional pivot, and I have never even looked back. I have never re-considered my decisions. I have never had any regrets. The opportunities that arose from this big pivot have been endless and oh so rewarding! If you had asked me 10 years ago if I would be here today, I never would have seen it coming. The diagnosis of RA, and the challenges that came with it, forced me to challenge myself to new professional roles. That allowed me more scheduling flexibility, a healthier lifestyle, and to learn new things that I never would have learned otherwise. It really did all work out!

Everyone has an RA journey. Thanks for listening to mine! RA is going to change your life no matter what you do. Choose to stay in control of the change! My advice— Take the leap, make the change, and don't be afraid to pivot!

Marla Nolan

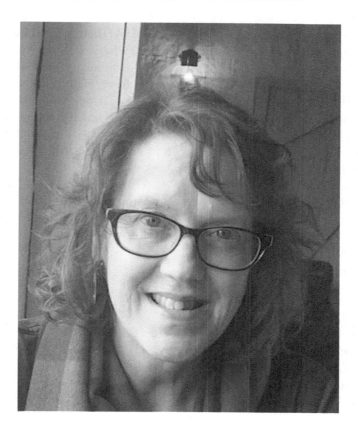

"What do we do? Do we give up? No! We adapt and find a new way to experience this wonderful life in spite of rheumatoid disease and limitations!"

As I wake up this morning, my jaw is painful and swollen near my ears, and I am unable to open my mouth to eat. It is 1989 and I am trying to finish up my graduate rotations for my pharmacy doctorate degree. I can hardly get dressed because my hand is so swollen, so I wrap it in ice and drive to work, because I am the pharmacy manager and I never call in sick. It is 1995. Home from work now, I go straight to the refrigerator for two bags of peas to place on my swollen knees and fall onto the couch to ice them. My step counter says I went seven miles at work today; it is 2001. "Just let me rest a bit," I say. I am laying on the floor in the independent pharmacy I own, from the fatigue that has overtaken my day. It is 2005. Feeling faint from the pain shooting down my legs from my back, I use a counter to catch my fall. I am now a regional pharmacy manager, visiting one of my 33 store teams, and my life is falling apart. I somehow drive myself home after finishing my day and call my husband to help me get into the house from the car. It is 2015 and this is my day every day. I am waving the white flag for help at my rheumatologist's office, and she places me on disability. This is a life lived with severe rheumatoid disease.

Deep depression and anxiety hit. How would we survive financially? I was only 53 and had planned to work until at least 60! I am so scared of what's going on with my body now. Usually, flares subside but not this one. Unfortunately, I learned I need major back surgery. I am sure that will fix everything, and I can go back to work after that. My rheumatoid disease had other ideas and continued to rage until I was utterly and completely "screeched to a halt."

Today at 60 years old, I am permanently disabled, and the long time pharmacist is now on chronic pain management, with few medication options left due to side effects. 33 years with my companion rheumatoid arthritis. So much loss. I used to be a distance runner, play piano, do cross stitch, hike, camp, go to six thrift stores in a day, visit my kids, etc. Now making dinner is an event and I often can't drive from the need of pain medication.

So, what do we do? Do we give up? No. We grieve, we cry, we scream, we get counseling, we find ways to adapt, and we find other ways to "be" in the world. And we realize this wonderful life continues to go on and is worth living.

In 2019, I decided to take a watercolor class that was online. It allowed me to work at my own slow pace by watching pre-recorded lessons. It was perfect because I could watch a bit from my recliner or bed, and paint a bit when I felt up to it. What I found was an incredible discovery. During the time that I refocused my mind from dealing with pain, fatigue, and depression, to watching beautiful pigment flow in water in beautiful ways on the paper, I had a little respite. Relief from my disabilities and pain. So, I watched YouTube, bought books to learn about painting and art, took more online classes and kept painting. I found that I could hold a brush in my deformed hands and create beauty which is ironic as I can't hold a glass anymore. I go to a meditative healing place when I am painting. We've converted a spare bedroom into a studio for me in our home, and I always have that special place I can go. It has helped me cope with the burden of chronic illness at this stage of my life.

The pivot from pharmacist to artist is something meaningful I can still do, and my disease cannot take it away from me. Did you know the famous oil painter Renior had rheumatoid arthritis and painted his whole life? I plan to as well. I have a website now, Marla Nolan Fine Art, where I sell my work and I donate a portion of my sales to the Arthritis Foundation. I also have a blog there, where I talk about being a disabled artist and the benefits of painting in chronic illness. I can't drive myself to work, stand or sit for very long at a time, punch a clock to work a full day, and can't hardly open anything anymore. But I can paint a little bit most days, mostly in pajamas and sometimes outside in the fresh air. And that makes me happy.

I hope my story will inspire you to try painting or some other form of art, as a part of your therapy plan to feel better. I hope you'll let me know if you do!

Saimun Singla

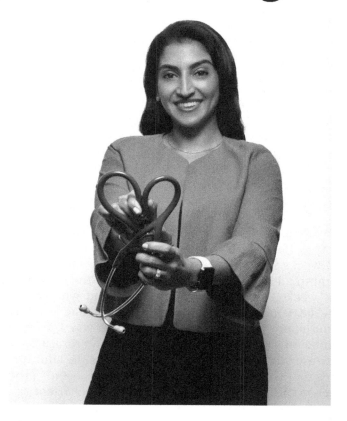

"When the doctor becomes a patient. How rheumatoid arthritis changed this pediatric rheumatologist's doctoring and career path."

For me, rheumatoid arthritis has been both a burden and benefit. Why on earth would I view this chronic illness with any ounce of positivity? Because as a physician myself, it gave me the gift of perspective that no medical training could have given me. When the doctor becomes a patient (of their own expertise nonetheless), treatment paradigms shift, and you begin to recognize the shortcomings of our current medical system--and how I as a physician fed into it.

Rheumatoid arthritis changed the trajectory of my career in a direction that I never imagined. My experience on the other side of the exam table allowed me to see that I was living and practicing in a "sick care model," where there was a pill or specialist for every complaint, that my choice of

words could be incredibly influential in helping patients handle their diagnosis, and that for a curious patient, most physicians are uninformed, or unaware of therapies past conventional treatment options.

The rheumatologist, who initially diagnosed me, explained that my diagnosis was "run-of-the-mill" in the world of rheumatology. Maybe she used this specific phrase because she was speaking to me as a colleague rather than a patient, but the wording left me feeling like I was a walking disease, not a person who had a disease. I thought about this experience for weeks.

Then I suddenly realized that it wasn't my doctor's fault. Throughout our medical training, we never studied people. Instead, we compulsively studied the pathology of disease, their treatments, mechanisms, and side effects. Patients were just bodies where a disease could manifest. Then I thought of how many times I unknowingly made a patient feel this way, and I became squeamish. That experience changed the way I interacted with my patients and their families. I began to listen more and became ultra-aware of my word choices.

My work at a large, tertiary care children's hospital, required mental and physical resiliency. This is nothing new in medicine. We are trained to be machines that won't quit unless absolutely necessary. There is no course on resilience, it's simply understood by all who enter the field. Imagine my annoyance when I realized that my arthritis was triggered by a critical aspect of my work as a physician--being on call in the hospital for the truly sick patients. Call required me to be available 24 hours a day, 7 days a week for a week at a time. Between my colleagues and I, we took turns covering the 52 weeks in a year. Every time I was woken up at night to address a question or concern during my call week, I woke up with stiffness in my fingers the next morning (taking hours to resolve). It took me many years to make the connection, but I would be on call, have a flare of my arthritis, be on high dose steroids for weeks afterwards, work hard to regain disease remission, and flare again after another week of being on call. I wanted this vicious cycle to stop. I knew what it would require--accommodations in writing from my rheumatologist to my boss. In my mind, this was the dreaded pinnacle of when one's diagnosis bleeds into their work life.

For a hardworking people-pleaser, this was uncomfortable, and left me feeling "less than" my colleagues, who were able to take hospital calls without bodily repercussions. In retrospect, if I would have stayed silent, was I really fulfilling the role of a resilient physician? By definition, resilient people "bounce back," psychologically and physically after challenges. This was the exact opposite of what I was doing prior to asking for accommodations. I wasn't "bouncing" back, I was trying to stay afloat so that I could function. In this scenario, the unspoken rules of my medical training served as a hindrance rather than help and required a large shift in mind-set to preserve my health.

The connection between stress, sleep deprivation, and disease flares wasn't a topic covered during medical school, residency, or fellowship training. Or that diet can play a role in disease activity, or that acupuncture might relieve joint pains, or that your social support and mental health are as important as taking your medications. The gaps in knowledge that conventional medicine left unanswered, led me to pursue additional training in integrative medicine--a specialty where I learned to blend conventional medicine with evidence-based complementary therapies. This training inspired me to pivot my career in a new direction, one that required leaving the long-term comfort and safety of my job in academia. In 2021, I left my position as an assistant professor at a top children's hospital and founded my own medical practice in Houston, named Rheum to Grow, for children with rheumatic conditions.

Here I practice medicine on my own terms, with a whole person approach that I think patients and families dealing with chronic illness deserve. It's critical that patients know their disease may be "run-of-the-mill," but that they themselves are not. At Rheum to Grow, I not only get to know a child's disease, but who they are as a person, what makes them flare, and what helps their symptoms. I get to doctor the way I would like to be treated, as if I were a patient there. Lucky for me, I know exactly what this entails. In addition to the use of labs, imaging, medications, and procedures, I address various factors that affect a child's health—the often-overlooked areas that can aggravate or alleviate rheumatic diseases. These include their nutrition patterns, exercise, sleep, stress, environment, emotional/self-regulatory abilities, resilience, and social support. My goal is to teach them that they can live and thrive with a chronic illness.

Rheumatoid arthritis has given me insight into being a patient--the person who must learn to navigate a complex healthcare system, personal life, and work to create a "new normal"—the body and life that awaits post-diagnosis. Although this condition has affected every part of my life, I am grateful to it. Because in the end, where would I be without it? I would have never taken that moment to reflect on my word choices in communicating with families, learned how to articulate my needs without feeling guilty, pursued additional fellowship training, or opened my own practice.

I've had many great mentors throughout my medical training, but this illness is by far the greatest one. My journey and experiences with rheumatoid arthritis, both good and bad, have served as advantages for me, because quite literally, it has given me a taste of my own medicine.

Shelley Fritz

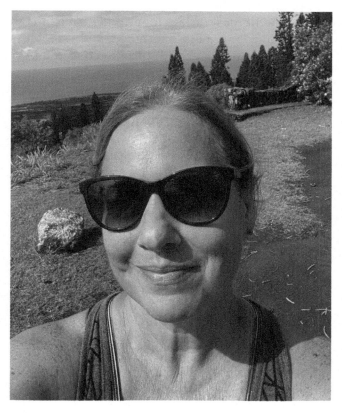

"My career as a teacher was rewarding, but it was also physically, mentally, and emotionally demanding, leading to exhaustion, stress, inflammation, and pain. Running away felt amazing, but hitting the reset button didn't produce instant results."

I'd do just about anything to feel better. So when the opportunity came up to quit my 25-year teaching career, and move from Florida to Hawaii, I took it. Friends and relatives have asked me if I feel better now that I live here. They wonder if my pain is gone in my serene environment. The short answer is no. With rheumatoid arthritis, fibromyalgia and osteoarthritis combined, I still have daily pain and fatigue, but it is far less intense nowadays. Hawaii is a magical place, but there is no magic wand to wipe away the symptoms of arthritis. I do feel dramatically better than I did before moving, but it turns out that had little to do with moving to Hawaii. I made monumental changes in how I live with my chronic illnesses.

I was diagnosed with rheumatoid arthritis in 2012 at age 42. The diagnosis came after two years of pain, and being misdiagnosed by a variety of specialists who treated my symptoms individually rather than connect the dots. I've been experiencing daily joint pain since 2010. Trial and error with biologics began with enbrel and humira, followed by a very brief stint with actemra, which caused drug-induced lupus, followed by a longer and more worthwhile time with orencia, until one day when it just quit working. The decision to change biologics was extremely difficult and filled me with anxiety. It's always a dive into the unknown, a giant leap of faith, that this will be the one that will be better than the last. Leaving work for infusions at the clinic meant missing at least a half day of work. Seeing how the list of biologics was dwindling, I looked to xeljanz, which I could take at home. I stayed on xeljanz for a little over a year until respiratory problems landed me in the hospital with pneumonia, pleurisy, and bilateral pulmonary embolisms. I'm always amazed at how casually I say that, but in reality, I almost died in April of 2017. Doctors could never pinpoint exactly what caused my PEs, although most blamed it on birth control. I spent six months on a blood thinner and I'm on baby aspirin for life. After a mandatory six month hiatus without RA meds, my doctors said JAK-inhibitors were no longer an option for me. Rituxan was in a different classification of drugs but this last biologic, on the list the doctor gave me, now became my greatest hope to feel better. Our relationship lasted a little over three years. Pile on the use of steroids and other meds like methotrexate, diclofenac, meloxicam, sulfasalazine, gabapentin, plaquenil, duloxetine, and prednisone over the last decade, and it's been a journey. Managing multiple chronic illnesses is like a full-time job in itself.

For years I daydreamed about stopping my stressful world from spinning. If I could quit my job and let my body dictate my schedule instead of a clock, my pain might diminish and maybe I might not need as many meds with side effects. As a teacher and professional development leader, I woke up before 5 a.m. on weekdays, and often on Saturdays, forced myself into the shower, struggled to put on clothes, then drove myself 45 minutes to work when my body screamed it wasn't ready yet. That morning routine played a game of ready-or-not with my body. With RA, my immune system attacks the synovium that lines my joints causing inflammation. Mornings are my most difficult part of the day due to soreness and stiffness. There were countless days when I cried in the shower over pain that made the simplest of tasks impossible. Since sitting for more than 15 minutes causes joint stiffness and muscle pain, long drives are very uncomfortable and often painful. My job required me to sit and stand for prolonged periods of time causing stiffness, and on days when fatigue was bad, I imagined curling up in a corner, so I loaded up on caffeine and comfort foods and pushed through the day. As the school bell rang, I prepped for more meetings and training that ran until sunset. I found myself using up all available energy, leaving me with nothing to give my family after the workday, then before I knew it, I was up again at the sound of the alarm clock. Things I loved in the past, like cooking dinner and spending time with friends and family, became stressful because I had extended myself too far with work, and not feeling strong enough to prepare dinner made me feel like I wasn't doing what I should be as a mother.

My career as a teacher was rewarding but it was also physically, mentally, and emotionally demanding, leading to exhaustion, stress, inflammation, and pain. While my mother was battling cancer in 2016, I stayed with her through the night then drove home to shower and change clothes to get to work by 7 a.m. That time would have been hard for anyone, but having RA and fibro made it even harder. Mom passed away in October 2016. The grief I felt losing my mother, whom I leaned on and spent time with daily, created a nonstop flare. I wasn't ready mentally or physically, but I went back to work.

This gravitational pull I had for my job seems so trivial now, but at the time it commandeered my focus and helped me compartmentalize my grief and pain. Work became increasingly challenging as my medicines failed to provide me enough relief. Constant pain, fatigue, and sleepless nights from "painsomnia" produced brain fog. I became forgetful, maybe unreliable at times, and my expectations for myself were greater than that, so I became overwhelmed with grief and depressed. I started blaming myself for my failures to accomplish all of my goals.

The cycle continued for three more years, until one day when I decided enough was enough. My husband accepted a job offer in Kauai, Hawaii, so I made the decision to retire from teaching after 25 years, pack my things, and move from Florida to Hawaii for a grandiose reset. Running away from the madness felt amazing, but hitting the reset button didn't produce instant results. I had to find a new medical team and jump over hurdles in a new insurance plan. My new rheumatologist and I discussed how my inflammation markers were high and my joint pain was worse. He suggested switching my biologic in hopes of lowering inflammation and disease activity. He proposed I go back to a TNF-blocker and take inflectra (iInfliximab), which is a biosimilar for remicade. My knowledge of biosimilars was limited so I did a lot of research and learned that inflectra is also used to treat conditions like ulcerative colitis and Crohn's, so with my gastrointestinal issues, this could be a good fit for decreasing inflammation.

Inflectra has worked better than any other drug I've tried. Side effects from NSAIDs and methotrexate resulted in bile acid malabsorption, microscopic colitis, and liver issues. My latest diagnoses were catalysts to stop eating my feelings, and to implement intentional weight loss through eating low inflammatory foods and exercising every day. I began with a two week reset by eating raw foods and eliminating my known triggers, like dairy and gluten, and potential triggers like sugar, processed foods, and red meat. I brought back in meat and sugar from natural sources like fruits, agave, and honey. I focused on moderation and because I wasn't on a rigid schedule, I was able to take time to build salads and cook using recipes that fit my needs. I cherish my morning one hour nature walks. They've become my personal time to reflect and absorb the beauty of the trees and birds around me. The most essential component of my plan has been removing the stress of continuous deadlines and late nights working. Retiring early, to be able to work flexibly, was the best decision for my body. Moving to a vacation spot is just the icing on the cake.

Over two years since moving, my pain is still present every day, but it's not as intense. The root of the problem is the physical toll it was taking on my body to be up and running, when it required a malleable schedule. I don't think I needed to move away to Hawaii to make my life less stressful. Had I stayed in Florida, I could have minimized stress, but I would have needed to make the same changes such as working remotely or with flexible hours. I would have needed to make serious lifestyle changes, with intentional focus on eating mostly unprocessed foods, to be able to control the inflammation in my gut, and I would have needed to minimize stress with daily exercise I enjoy. I've spent 10 years fighting with RA, OA, and fibro, while trying to make peace with myself and I'm finally getting closer to finding that peace.

Molly Overkamp

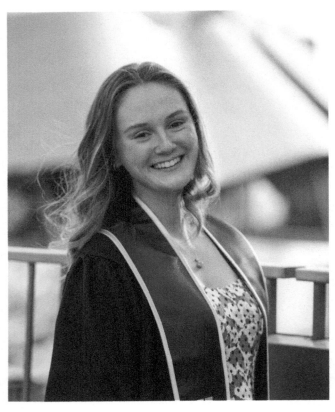

"I can only hope that the practice of overworking employees begins to dissipate, so more disabled people can feel comfortable working within the system they spend so much time interacting with for their own health."

About a year before I began developing arthritis symptoms, I started a new job at a mental health group home. I had just turned twenty and was trying to find new experiences that would help me decide what career path I wanted to pursue. I had never worked in mental health before, and so I followed the ethical guidelines given to me by the company, and didn't give much critical thought to the ideas at the time.

One very important point the company emphasized was that these clients were opening their home to new hires, they were allowing total strangers to learn about the most challenging parts of their life, manage their healthcare, and help them make decisions regarding their wellbeing. Understanding the gravity of the role, I set boundaries with clients according to company policy; the complications of my life — health, family, relationships — were not of the client's concern. It was important not to give reason for anxiety, especially when relationships, between employees and clients, were by their very nature transient. If an employee leaves the company, the clients' should not have information about the employee that would cause them to worry about that employee.

All of this meant that when I began to develop symptoms of what ended up being rheumatoid arthritis, I did my best to prevent my symptoms from seeping into my work. Of course, this was an unattainable goal; my knees were so swollen that my legs couldn't extend to the 180° required for me to stand up right. My job duties didn't allow me to hide my symptoms behind a desk, and the clients would stop me and inquire about how I was feeling. Because these were people that I had known for over a year now, I understood why they were curious — they cared for me as I cared for them. But I could not shake the feeling that I was failing them, that somehow my health crisis was making their health worse. I would hear the voice of the training modules in my head, admonishing me for not maintaining work-life boundaries. And so every time a client stopped to ask me what was wrong, I just answered that I was, *"just a little stiff"* and, *"it's nothing to worry about."*

That line quickly became unconvincing; in addition to struggling to walk and climb stairs, I now struggled to open medication bottles, write notes, or pour coffee. When I served meals, my hands shook and I often dropped utensils, plates, and food. I was losing a lot of weight, and clients began to point out that my clothes weren't fitting as well. With all visual evidence indicating the contrary, saying *"I was just a little stiff,"* left my clients looking at me dumbfounded. But even as my personal life was crumbling in the face of my illness, I maintained the facade at work, thinking that it was in the clients' best interest.

Outside of my relationships with clients, the quality of my work was suffering. Prior to arthritis, I was considered an anchor of the office. I had worked at the home for longer than most of the other part-time staff and could finish quite a bit of important tasks during my two shifts per week.

But arthritis made it feel like I was moving in slow motion; sending emails, organizing the medication cart, and doing client rounds, took me three times as long as it did before my diagnosis. I sat in front of my colleagues during shift-change, feeling defeated as I told them all of the tasks that I hadn't gotten a chance to finish.

As my disease continued to worsen, I felt more and more exhausted at the end of every shift. The medications I was taking made me feel nauseous, and I could barely eat any of the food I had packed for work. After my shift, I would collapse in bed with my work clothes still on. I would wake up in the morning, having slept for nearly twelve hours, feeling as though I had run a marathon without any training.

One night towards the end of October, I went to work dressed in my Halloween costume. Holidays at work were often a morale booster for employees and clients alike. Given that it was a special occasion, I put a lot of effort into planning my costume despite my declining health. The evening was spent eating candy with clients and watching scary movies, but inside I was feeling more nauseous than ever before. I was so hungry, but no matter how much I ate, I wasn't satiated. I sat in the office, feeling faint and wondering if I could safely walk to my car without falling. I remained in the office for nearly an hour after my shift chatting with the overnight staff, all the while trying to muster up the strength to pack up my things, walk down the block to my car, and take the thirty minute drive back to my house. I didn't know that I had just worked my last shift at that job.

When I woke up the next morning, I had 105°F fever and was advised by a 24 hour nurse line to head to the emergency room. It was a Sunday, and luckily the ER was fairly empty. My fever broke after they gave me some Tylenol and saline via IV, and they sent me home. But the fever returned and pretty soon I was limping into the urgency clinic at my university. After two hours of bouncing back and forth to different observation rooms, I sat weary-eyed on a bed in the doctor's office as I listened to him explain to me that I was actually allergic to the medication I had been taking. My liver had developed hepatitis from the drug, and would require high-dose prednisone for at least a month to help my liver recover. For whatever reason, it was at that moment I finally realized the way I was living was unsustainable. I had been ignoring the effects of arthritis, and it had finally caught up with me.

I went home and called my boss to tell her what had happened. Due to the nature of my job, it wasn't feasible for me to leave for an undetermined amount of time. I had no idea when I would be fit to work again, so I ended up having to quit, effective immediately. I was crushed — here I was, having deteriorated before my clients' very eyes, and now I had effectively disappeared without being able to give them any explanation. All of my efforts to prevent them from worrying had been in vain, and I didn't even get the chance to say goodbye. And now I was unemployed for the first time since I turned 16. I was graduating from college in the coming months and couldn't even hope to begin post-grad life with all of my friends. I spent my month recovering from hepatitis crying for all that I had lost.

I was lucky to be able to visit the group home one last time after that month was over. I got to sit with the clients without having to think about anything work-related; I just sat and visited for hours. The obligations of maintaining boundaries rang loudly in my ears, but I did my best to ignore it. After all, many of these clients had their plans derailed due to illness. Of all the people in this world, these were the people who would understand what I was going through. They deserved honesty, and so I gave it to them. After the visit, I left finally feeling ready to focus on my health and let the grief from closing this chapter of my life go.

Five months later, I am still without medication that works and am still unemployed. I'm grateful to live with my parents and be on their health insurance plan, but I want to gain independence and start a career in healthcare. Once I'm able to work, I worry I'll have to quit the moment I experience any health complications. "Grind" culture is so ingrained in the healthcare field, and I fear I will be ostracized at work if I ask for accommodations. I can only hope that the practice of overworking employees begins to dissipate, so more disabled people can feel comfortable working within the system they spend so much time interacting with for their own health. I wish I could end this short story by saying I found a job that accommodates me and makes me happy, but, the truth is, I am still at the point in my arthritis journey where so much is unknown and undecided. I am learning to live with the ambiguity of my future, and I find comfort in knowing that many people with arthritis eventually find relief and do amazing things. I know that will eventually be possible for me as well.

Stacy Arvin

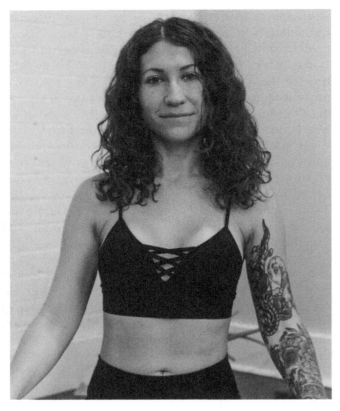

"With rheumatoid arthritis you are always going to be reminded of how this disease affects your life. Bruce Lee said, "Be water my friend." Be flexible in the mind, body and soul. Be open to change and let each new transition be part of your healing journey."

Born and raised in Middle Tennessee, I grew up mildly active and ate a typical southern diet, high carbs, saturated fats and processed sugar. My activity of choice was dance! I loved music, costumes, fashion and performing! As I grew older, I was participating in three to five dance classes per week, while still supporting my body with a southern fried diet. Without knowing it, I was already maxing out at a young age, based on nutrition alone. I was forced to cut my dancing career short, due to repeated knee injuries, not rehabilitating properly and I decided to move forward with some of my other interests.

In August of 2008, I started my senior year of high school ready to graduate and start my cosmetology career at Paul Mitchell, the School of Nashville. My plan was to become a five-star stylist in Nashville. The school year hadn't started yet and I began having strange pains in my feet, like my shoes were a size too small. Pain then spread to my ankle, making it impossible for me to walk - then to my hands, to the point of not being able to open doors. After many doctor visits and tons of testing, all before my 18th birthday, I was diagnosed with rheumatoid arthritis.

At my first follow up appointment, after finally being diagnosed, a doctor and I discussed my future and possible options for medication. To my surprise, I was laughed at when I said I was going to cosmetology school to be a stylist. I couldn't believe a medical professional, who I was looking to for advice on my health, laughed at me instead of helping me! At this point, I knew it would be a long journey. I also learned quickly that I'd need to be my biggest advocate and fight to prove everyone wrong.

I grew up with a homeopathic approach to medicine, so I was nervous about the medications offered to me. The most effective drugs were injections, which was my last resort, so I started with pill options. I went through over five doctors, and many different steroids/pills for pain relief, but nothing was helping. I had to turn to the injections. I finally started to feel some relief but the side effects always made me question if this was truly the best option for me.

Fast forward a few years. I'm now 25 years old and managing a five-star salon, working 10+ hour shifts/five days a week, while sometimes seeing up to 10 people a day! Everyone can relate to the stress this puts on us, mentally and physically. At this point, I had been on antidepressant/anxiety medication for 10 years, thyroid medication for four years and using the injections for almost five years (with the benefits slowly wearing out). On a pain scale of 1-10, I was working day-to-day with joint pain at level eight, just trying to find energy to search for other options.

Remission from RA. is less than 30% likely but I desired any kind of control over my health. I had been conditioned to think that I couldn't change and it bothered me deep down to my core. To think

I would have to rely on medication the rest of my life was something I couldn't live with so I started focusing on what else I could do for myself. It was time to put myself first in a career where I'd always put my clients' needs before mine.

It wasn't an easy process. My boss at the time had seen me working my hardest, but I was overworking my body. Explaining to her that I could no longer work the same schedule, because of my body's pain, didn't make sense to her since she never heard me complain or saw me grimace. I never complained. How can you expect your clientele to grow when you're explaining to them what you're dealing with? I stepped down from managing, cut back my hours and stopped double booking clients. I started practicing yoga daily to keep my body moving, meditating to ease my mind and, most importantly, finally decided to change my diet.

I'd taken a food allergy test before and had done tons of personal research on plant based diets but wasn't committed to making that change yet. I'd read stories of people coming off of major medications by going plant based. My medicine had been slowly wearing off so I hadn't had an injection for three weeks. I thought then would be the time to see if an all plant based diet would help me. Within 24 hours, my overall pain immediately went from level eight to level three. For the first time in a while, I felt good! I continued this until my next scheduled appointment with my physician specialist for blood work and x-Rays. After my appointment, I received a phone call from the specialist's office updating me with my test results. She said, sort of surprisingly, *"Everything looks great. I see no additional joint damage. Continue following your plant based diet and let's monitor this every six months."*

She was the first doctor to encourage these dietary changes, and help monitor my progress to assure this was the best option for me. I wanted to know more! What else could I do to take care of my health?

I believe that what goes on your body is just as important as what goes in your body! I started to dig into salons that only use non-toxic products, and why stylists were making that switch. Some stylists were feeling relief from joint pain, while most stylists experienced fewer headaches, and reduced skin irritation, after changing to a chemical-free environment. I knew this was another step for me to take. I left the salon I was managing and decided to move to Nashville to start creating my dreams. I began working as a contracted stylist at a non-toxic salon and gained more control over my schedule. I went from working eleven hour shifts, five days a week in a traditional salon to working six hour shifts, three days a week in a non-toxic and chemical-free salon environment.

A lot of things were different now. My paychecks weren't the same but my mind, body and soul were expanding in ways I never thought were possible. I now had free time to re-evaluate my life. I knew from day one of my cosmetology career that it was going to be limited. Since I had started, so much had changed for my body and I. Now I wanted to incorporate my healing journey. Soul work, fitness and nourishment choices were all a huge part. In the next two years, I grew my professional skills through continued education focusing on creating a business that I could grow old with. I became a reiki master, yoga instructor, certified personal trainer and certified plant based nutritionist.

It was time for me to shed the image I'd created for myself as a hairstylist. I was ready to share my personal experiences and professional knowledge with my clients, who had only seen me as a hairstylist for the past 10 years! In 2019, my husband and I started our creative lifestyle company, Style & Soul, LLC, and opened my own boutique spa salon on Nashville's Music Row in 2020. My salon spa, Blue Dream Salon, was focused on mind, body and soul rejuvenation while providing hair, skin, body and energy services. In 2021, we launched our plant based wellness brand, Dreamss Supplements. We created Blue Dream Salon to be an opportunity for retirement. In January of 2022, I began the transition of my cosmetology career, to a health and wellness career focused on healing the mind, body and soul. My technique and experience as a stylist and salon owner will live on through my successor.

I now share what I have learned along the way to help people who used to be like me; young people with tough questions that they can't find the answers for. Living with chronic pain and fatigue at a young age gave me a mental toughness comparable to Kobe's Mamba Mentality. A mental toughness that pushes me to overcome whatever life has thrown my way! I say all this to empower you and let you know that nothing can hold you back, only your mentality.

Sydney Foster

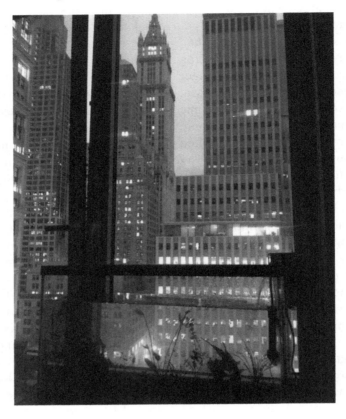

"Even being arthritic, I'm still a person just like anyone else and I can do things, even if it takes a little longer (and a slightly different route)."

As long as I can remember, I knew what I wanted to be when I grew up and what I was going to do with my life. I was going to work with horses. I would muck stalls and lift hay bales and communicate with half ton prey animals. Before I even knew what college was, I knew what school I wanted to go to and what I wanted to go for. I wanted to be a stablehand, and maybe, just maybe, have my own barn someday. My family couldn't always afford lessons, so any experience I could have with horses, I jumped upon. There was a therapy barn near where I lived, you could volunteer to be a stablehand, but you had to be 13, so I counted down the days. The first few years went great. During the summer I was in more often than a good portion of the staff. I loved it so much my sister even joined in for a bit. But then,

at the start of what would be my third summer, my knees began to hurt, my shoulders too, my grip was weaker, among other things. I assumed I was out of shape, but as the summer went on and my body failed to adjust as it had in the years prior, I thought something may be up.

I went to the doctor, who told me it was growing pains, then my weight, etc. When my symptoms didn't stop after I clearly wasn't going to grow, and had lost weight but felt worse, he sent me to a rheumatologist. It turns out that I had lyme disease, and as a result, lyme arthritis. After finding out what lyme disease was, I realized the cruel twist of fate that had been thrust upon me, my love of horses was going to prevent me from my dreams of a career with them. I decided that I was stronger than lyme, but I continued to get worse.

The summer before my senior year, what would be my fourth summer at the barn. I realized that it was too dangerous for me to be in a barn in my current state of health. It was soon after that I realized that my plans for college, even my major, just wasn't possible. In looking through emails I got from colleges that year, I had a few fantasies about going to college in New York City, studying art, living in the big city, becoming an art therapist. After all, my dreams while working at the therapy barn had been to become an equine therapist, and somehow incorporate art into it. It didn't take me long to find a couple of schools that had everything I was looking for. I was able to visit both schools and at one I felt as though my future self was already living there, like I was destined to go there, and the other school wasn't all it was cracked up to be.

So come fall I applied to that college in NYC, and a backup, closer to home, just in case. I was accepted to both, and with some incredible scholarships that made college in NYC feasible. My family took me back to the school for a final visit and it only solidified my love. My family could hardly believe my quick change in tone. My previous dream school and major could hardly be more different. My top choice school had accepted me and it was time for me to accept them back. Suddenly, I couldn't wait to graduate and my thoughts of the future were no longer of the countryside, but the big city. As my senior year went on I got sicker, but I was not going to let anything dash my second chance. At orientation I made a friend who asked me to be his roommate. My life was like a fantasy, granted it was not the one I had planned, but the one I felt I was supposed to live. It was about a week into my anthropology class that I decided to switch majors to be an anthro/psych major, with an art minor as I got to discover who I was for the first time, while being introduced to so many new things.

I felt right at home in the big city, I figured out the subways, loved the crowds, found a park to call my study spot. My health was still deteriorating, but it felt like I was supposed to be there, and as I looked back I realized that I had no idea how I would have gotten to where I was without my arthritis. Then things took a bit of a turn once again. My roommate moved out and things began to fall apart, my grandma began calling me, nervous about this "Covid" thing that hadn't even hit the states yet (officially), my health got almost unbearable and my friends disappeared. While I still felt like I belonged to New York City, I made the decision that the coming semester would be my second and final semester at this college, as for now it wasn't the right time. I still loved my classes, they were the redeeming thing about that time. I even did projects for a political art class that helped my able bodied classmates understand what being disabled is like, and I am still proud of those projects today. Soon Covid hit the states and one week of missed classes turned to spring break being extended indefinitely.

At first my depression got worse, but then I started realizing that this is a chance to get the rest that my body desperately needed. I was able to work on art for myself in my time frame, rather than the school's quick deadlines. During that time I fell back in love with fiber arts. I had crocheted, as much as time and my health allowed, while at school, even tried to intertwine it with my classes, but my health issues and little free time prevailed. I had been crocheting since I was around seven and it has been a part of my life since, but not as big of a part as I felt it was supposed to be. After getting the rest I needed during 2020, I was revitalized in 2021. I was not cured, but it did not take as much of a toll on me when the furthest I needed to go was up or down 11 stairs. I was able to dedicate much of my time and energy to crochet, and decided to open my own shop, though that continues to be postponed.

As the lockdowns went away I got a job, which has slowed my production down. I was able to be way more in tune with my body for around 18 months. I may not be able to crochet as fast as an able bodied artist, my art is unique to me and allows me to express myself. Since I stepped away from school and traditional jobs, I have figured out that I do love city life, psychology and helping people, but I do not want fine arts to be my main career. I hope to be a forensic psychologist and for now I'm an entrepreneur and small business owner, several words I never would have ever thought I'd be able to call myself. I'm still riding the highs and lows of life, but I'm getting better and realizing that even being arthritic, I'm still a person just like anyone else and I can do things, even if it takes a little longer (and a slightly different route). I haven't given up on working with horses, recently I've been feeling better. I even got back to the barn I had volunteered at before, it turns out several of the horses have lyme disease too.

Julie Bastarache

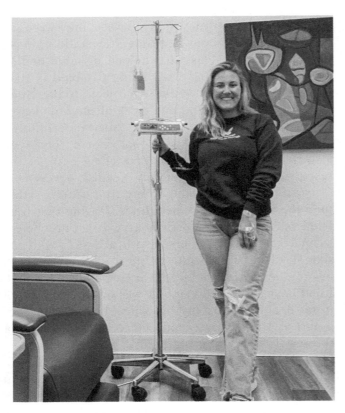

"Arthritis: people don't "get it" until they get it."

I'm originally from the Maritime. I moved to Ottawa to pursue my studies and became a dental hygienist. Unfortunately, only two short years after I graduated, I got diagnosed with rheumatoid arthritis which brought a halt to my career. My health was deteriorating quicker than I had hoped and so I had to make the difficult decision to hang up my scrubs and scaling instruments. I now work as a treatment coordinator for a group of oral and maxillo-facial surgeons here in the city.

I started my Instagram account, The Healing Spoonie shortly after my diagnosis in 2019, in hopes of finding other folks living through the same (or similar) thing as me, because if you have a chronic illness, you know that people don't "get it" until they get it. Almost three years later, there are now over 1600 of you following along! Thank you all for being here, and I hope that I can shed light on what it's like living with an incurable illness.

A few fun arthritis facts:

- Six million Canadians have a form of arthritis - that's one in five!!
- Over half of people with arthritis are UNDER the age of 65. Yup you read that right; arthritis is not just an "old person's disease."
- Arthritis is a complex disease with over 100 different types. The most common being osteoarthritis (wear and tear of the joints).
- Inflammatory arthritis also comes in different types such as rheumatoid arthritis (RA), childhood arthritis (or JIA), psoriatic arthritis (PsA), ankylosing spondylitis (AS), etc.
- Many drugs used to treat inflammatory arthritis require a "wash out" period before considering trying to conceive.
- People living with arthritis are more likely to develop anxiety, mood disorders, poor mental health, and difficulty sleeping (painsomnia).
- Trying to find a medicine regime that works is like trial and error. Many drugs require months to fully take effect, and you won't know if it's working (or not) until you've been on them for a certain period of time. I'm three years into this and still haven't found a combination that makes me feel good.
- Trying to get coverage for the (very) expensive drugs is half of the battle! Insurance companies want to make sure you've tried all the other least expensive options before they consider covering you for the drugs that actually work (step therapy) - because of course, some random insurance clerk knows your health better than you and your doctor.

Suffice to say, if you live with a chronic illness such as arthritis, you are not alone. New diagnoses can be scary, but it's important to speak up and raise awareness so that less people live feeling like they are the only one.

Brianna Brade

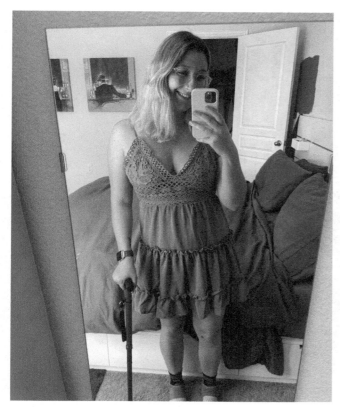

"Exploring the freedom of adapting lifestyles and putting yourself above your career."

I have always been career-oriented and advancement in my field was one of my top priorities. I put so much weight on myself to excel and never let life get in the way of my goals. Some may see that as a fault but it was the way I had always been, and I thrived in a fast-paced environment. I loved school, worked full-time to put myself through college and worked my way up the corporate ladder. However, I was eight months into my dream role when I started to get sick. This was not a sickness I could push through. I didn't understand. I had never faced an obstacle that touched every portion of my daily life. I did my best to manage my health and company expectations, going through diagnosis and treatment with accommodations. As each week went by, I became more unhappy with my situation. It felt as though I was failing, not only as an employee but as a person. I did not know how to cope with illness directly impacting my ability to do what I loved. However, as time went on I started to realize that I did not value this role over my health, neither physical or mental. A shift was happening within me and eventually, I embraced it.

I resigned from my role three months after my ankylosing spondylitis (AS) diagnosis, the battle had gone on long enough. Between the PT, injections, daily medications and symptoms, my life had to shift to prioritizing health. The weight of the diagnosis alone was soul-crushing. I was in my early 20s and had only been in my field for four years. It didn't feel fair but that's the thing -- we will always be faced with unpredictability and if we do not adapt, we will not overcome. Choosing my health over my work was a weight off my shoulders, which surprised me considering the turmoil I had gone through over the decision. I realized that this role was not conducive with my health, and I could surely find work that better fit my needs. I am hopeful in continuing my path remotely and encourage anyone struggling with their line of work to look at all their options, as adjustments can be made

Since putting my health first, I have found my mental space is significantly clearer. I couldn't believe how freeing it was to be able to remove myself from a, now toxic, work environment. I know everyone doesn't have the privilege to leave their job but I encourage you to try to put your health first, as our bodies and minds are much more important than commuting downtown every day.

Julia Walker

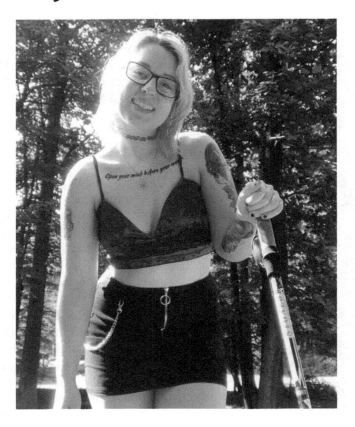

"This isn't a story with a happy ending. And there won't ever be a happy ending unless we completely reform social security and disability benefits."

My arthritis story began in high school. I was a varsity athlete, an honors/AP student, and a band geek. I even juggled two part time jobs in addition to my school activities. Everything changed during my junior year of high school. I was 16, and it was fall. While I didn't know it at the time, my body had already started declining. My sophomore year, I was number four on varsity. Everyone expected me to be number one my junior and senior year. I wanted to apply to colleges on sports scholarships and dreamed of playing in national tennis leagues.

That year I ended up being thrown all the way back to number nine. Typically there would only be eight varsity players, but they kept me as a second alternate, so I wouldn't have to go down to junior varsity and away from my friends. My mental health hadn't been doing so great either, so I just chalked it up to that. After all, tennis is half physical, half mental. But little did I know that it was both my physical and mental health that caused the decline in my skills. At the end of the season, I thought I had a stress fracture. Turns out, that was the beginning of my journey with rheumatoid arthritis. Since then, I've been on a handful of different medications, just so I can live life somewhat comfortably.

Most of my life growing up as a child I wanted to work in medicine. I wanted to be a dentist, a pediatrician, a surgeon, an immunologist, I wanted to do research and so much more. But my RA affected my hands a lot at first, and even just writing with a pencil was painful. I knew that doing things like research and working in a lab wouldn't be safe. My hands are weak and I'm clumsy. That would be a huge safety hazard. And forget about working on patients. I wouldn't be able to do stitches without my tremors getting in the way.

During my senior year of high school, I decided to start looking into college for music business and marketing. I thought that working in live music and festivals would be easier for me, especially because I wouldn't have to go to school for as long, and I wouldn't be responsible for patients or anyone except for myself. Throughout college I worked a few music festivals, and even landed a gig doing social media marketing for a local music venue. Unfortunately that was cut short due to the pandemic. And now, two years later, I've realized that working in the live music industry just wouldn't be feasible. The last concert I went to before Covid, I almost left early because I was in so much pain from standing.

My illnesses have gotten worse, and I've been diagnosed with gerd, gastroparesis, and dysautonomia along with my rheumatoid arthritis. I've had unknown neurological issues and muscle weakness. Nowadays I work a minimum wage job from home. The pay isn't much and I don't have benefits. I'm terrified for when I turn 26 and can no longer be on my parents insurance. I am incredibly fortunate for the job that I have. It works with my illnesses and I was able to get accommodations with a special keyboard and mouse for my hands.

I'm currently 24 years old. I have less than two years to find a job that works with my disabilities and also has good health insurance. I know that if I have to end up on medicaid through the government, my health will deteriorate. I won't be able to afford the medications that keep me somewhat functioning. This isn't a story with a happy ending. And there won't ever be a happy ending unless we completely reform social security and disability benefits. Being disabled and having rheumatoid arthritis isn't so bad when the right accommodations, tools and support are available. But I will always be fearful of the future whilst grieving what could have been.

In my spare time, I raise awareness for rheumatoid arthritis and my other comorbidities online. TikTok and Instagram have really helped me find a community of people just like me, and I've even been able to make some money off of surveys I've found through TikTok. Advocating for myself and disabled people has become a huge passion of mine, and it brings me a lot of joy. I've even been able to share some of what I've learned with my coworkers, so that whenever we have a customer that is disabled they know what to do. I'm super grateful for social media. The disability community is full of so many amazing people, all trying to make the world a better place. If you'd like to follow, my usernames on Instagram and TikTok are dynamicallydisabled. Thank you for reading my story!

Tracy Augustine

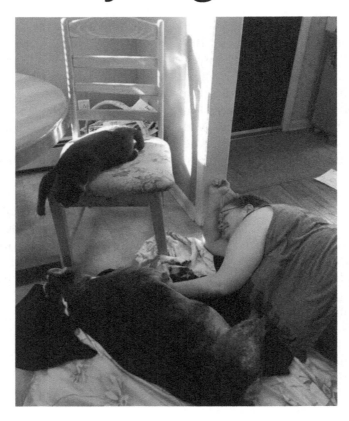

"If I never got sick, I would have never learned that you must be relentless when pursuing a medical diagnosis."

What If I Never Got Sick With Arthritis

In 2009 I was ripped out of my life of working 50 hours a week, being able-bodied, and living life like a typical 25 year old. Overnight, I went from being healthy to laying in a hospital bed unable to move because I was in unbearable pain. I was diagnosed with rheumatoid arthritis, fibromyalgia, and knee osteoarthritis. The last 13 years have been a never-ending list of medical problems related to my arthritis, multiple orthopedic surgeries, joint pain, and fatigue that keeps me in bed for days. My mental health suffered from getting very sick very quickly. I was lost trying to live this new life full of hospital stays and medical appointments. It is easy to lose perspective on the good things

when you experience a life changing medical crisis. After living with arthritis for 10 years, I started to have a better outlook; I had access to the medicine that would change the trajectory of my disease. I was able to assemble an amazing medical team full of compassionate providers. On the 10th anniversary of the onset of my arthritis, (I lovingly call this day my sick-iversary), I made a list of all the positive things my arthritis brought into my life.

If I never got sick, I would have continued to work 50-60 hours a week and not been available to my friends and family. I was always too busy for them because work came first. Getting sick forced me to slow down. Now I have all the time in the world to be there for people in need.

If I never got sick, I would have never learned to stand up for myself. When the wrong doctors gave me the wrong diagnosis, even when I was clearly suffering, it was earth shattering. I found a strength I never knew I had to fight for myself.

If I never got sick, I would have never learned to appreciate rest. My body betrayed me and shut down. I have learned that rest is vital. I schedule days where all I do is rest. It has become a priority for me.

If I never got sick, I would have never come to God. Sickness took away all the plans I had for my life. But God showed me the plans that He has for me. My kingdom needed to fall for me to join His.

If I never got sick, I would have never had the time to volunteer at a cat rescue where I met my cat, Hannah. The moment she jumped out of the cage and into my arms, I knew she was mine. She keeps me anchored to this world.

If I never got sick, I would have never learned that you must be relentless when pursuing a medical diagnosis. For three years I had rheumatologists who didn't believe me when I told them how much pain I was in. I learned to never, ever give up when seeking a diagnosis or the latest treatments. When I finally found my dream rheumatologist, it felt like a huge weight lifted off my chest. I had hope for the first time in five years.

If I never got sick, I wouldn't have been able to take care of my dog, Casey as she was dying from cancer. It would have been torture for me to go to work while she was sick. Casey was (and still is) my soulmate. She always knew when I was having a difficult day. When my hands or my knees were swollen, she instinctively knew and would lick them for the ultimate source of moist heat. When she was diagnosed with cancer, the vet told us she had two months to live. I committed myself to staying home with her and taking care of her. She lived for eight months, which was a miracle. She died the day after my second arthritis advocacy event. I think she knew I had this amazing support system. I can picture her saying "this is where I leave you. You have people now." I still deal with the grief of losing her every day, but I am grateful I was able to spend the last months of her life with her.

If I never got sick, I would have never met my arthritis family. They are my tribe. These people show up for me. They understand my pain in ways no one else can. They have quickly become my family. Recently, I was daydreaming what my life would be like if I never got sick. I was getting lost in a dream world of being able-bodied, having financial independence and doing all that I used to be able to do. Then something stopped me dead in my tracks. I realized if I never got sick, I would have never met these brave arthritis warriors. My life suddenly seemed so empty. It felt like the air got knocked out of my lungs. I am so blessed to have this amazing family.

If I never got sick, I would have never learned how to advocate. I was always too busy to help non-profits. I never had the time to learn how to advocate or get any training before I got sick. If you would have told me pre-2009 that I would be meeting with members of congress, I would have laughed at you. Meeting with legislators is something I would have never had the courage to do.

If I never got sick, I would have never started fundraising for my favorite arthritis non-profits. I have an annual fundraiser called Auction for Arthritis and a garage sale. In the last four years, I raised over $10,000. Planning these fundraisers allowed me to find purpose in my pain.

If I never got sick, I would have never met my arthritis mentor. My friend Kerry and I met at an arthritis advocacy event. I was instantly drawn to her warm heart and glowing personality. We kept in touch for a year and saw each other at a conference the following year. I can't explain why the subsequent events happened, but I started following her around the conference. I think I was just so happy to see Kerry and she was such an inspiration to me that I just wanted to soak up all the time I could get with her. I'm incredibly lucky that Kerry has a great sense of humor and took it all in stride. She is the only person I ask about event planning for fundraisers, and she always gives me the best advice. Kerry radiates positivity and does countless outreach and service for the arthritis community.

This list grows each year. I'm always finding new things to be grateful for with my arthritis. It is tangible proof that I came out on the other side of something that was meant to break me.

Elisa Comer

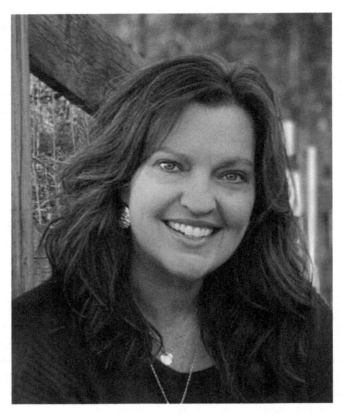

"My goals reside more within the realm of the intangibles these days. It's a never-ending discussion that goes back and forth, leaving a trail of broken dreams, unmet expectations and unachievable goals in its wake."

Just Five Seconds: When Chronic Illness Re-Sets our Goals

Five seconds..It was down in just five seconds. The huge, towering tree that we'd watched for almost 20 years was gone. The strong, tall tree that for over a decade had housed our beautiful red-tailed hawks and their babies, was lost to the terribly destructive disease of the ash borer beetle. Now weakened and unsafe, it literally took seconds for the tree removal company to take it down.

I was kind of sad, seeing it fall. We loved that tree. It was our tallest, so was part of the skyline during sunrises and sunsets on the farm. Later that day and into the evening, I watched as our hawks circled around and around overhead, wondering where their home had gone. They seemed to know that the landscape was different. The place they'd called home, their familiar place, their place of comfort, was no longer.

And it took just five seconds.

I live with rheumatoid arthritis. I was also diagnosed with Sjogrens syndrome and much later, myasthenia gravis. Just like the tree I reference above, life as I knew it changed dramatically when my health took a nosedive from chronic illness. How I would live, work, enjoy friendships, relate to family, everything as I knew it came tumbling down. Heck, even how I would brush my teeth changed.

Chronic illness is a game-changer. I always knew this, but until I actually experienced it personally, I didn't have the capacity to understand just how deeply chronic illness would affect life as I knew it. My sphere of comfort and routine would be turned inside out and goals, hopes, and dreams would come tumbling down in an instant. The pain, fatigue, brain fog, financial ruin (it's really expensive to be this dang sick), exhaustion, and inability to do the things I'd always done demanded a redefining of how I did life. You see, there's a collision between RA and mindset, a space where the mind and body collide. The mind says, *"this is what I want to do,"* and the body says, *"nope, not happening, not today."* It's a never-ending discussion that goes back and forth, leaving a trail of broken dreams, unmet expectations and unachievable goals in its wake.

One of these collisions happened when I was forced to quit work. I remember well when I had to leave the workforce, it's actually happened twice. The change from award-winning, well-known small business owner to staying home to be sick, and from re-entering the workforce as a worship leader, to staying home this time permanently, took a toll on my mind unlike anything the pain or fatigue would be able to cause. I even tried volunteering, but no one wanted to sign up someone who could never promise they'd be able to show up. I tried music endeavors, but a season of broken bones from the effects of RA left me unable to play my instrument. It became obvious that working, volunteering, and helping on any kind of predictable schedule wasn't in the cards for me neither in that moment, nor in moments to come.

That was my collision point, recognizing, *"nor in moments to come,"* as my new reality. After a long season of broken bones and subsequent surgeries, where I spent more time in the hospital or in a cast (or both) than out, I finally forced my hand on the one change I'd been avoiding, the one thing I did not want to do, the one thing that would indicate surrender to this horrible disease... I had to re-define my goals. I tried everything to avoid this step. Pushing through the pain. Doing things in small spurts. Making long days happen, knowing I'd crash for several days afterward, and just accepting it. But my body won. There's only so far you can push before you really do crash. Hospitalizations. Splints and casts. Surgeries. Inability to get out of bed on your own. Inability to use your hands, or even make a fist for that matter. Nobody can push through that, and there comes a time when it's just not smart to keep trying. In one of the collision moments, my goals - what I'd always wanted to do, what I'd hope to be able to achieve, the legacy I'd prayed to leave to those around me - came crashing down. And this time I knew it was for real. Permanent. It seemed to take just five seconds.

Nowadays, I live without the pressure of achievement. Like tall trees riddled with the disease of beetles and bugs, my old goals were overtaken by RA and the other diagnoses I had. Just like that tree, all my goals came tumbling down. Appropriately so, though I didn't believe it in the beginning. Re-defining goals, while oppressing at the time, is now something I find quite liberating. Often, no one requires that much of me except... well, me. Rheumatoid disease has forced this over-achiever, or perhaps more aptly called "achievement addict," to look to other things, deeper things, for what defines me than simply what I can achieve in a day. RA doesn't allow achievement to be a definition of much of anything. I guess "rest" can be an achievement, and some days this is all I can do, and intentional rest is something I still struggle with. Considering it as just another med on my list helps me appreciate its importance. My goals reside more within the realm of the intangibles these days. Being kind. Being generous. Giving my family first dibs on my energy tank. Making memories. Reaching out to others who live with chronic illness just like I do and sharing our wins, and even our losses, so that we know there are others who understand.

You see, my goals aren't gone, they're just different. Life threw me a huge curve and while I had to work through a long period of resistance, I've finally made progress on following this crazy road I'm on. Lots of hairpin curves, but I'm doing better at riding those, albeit quite slowly at times. I try to be in the driver's seat, but RA sometimes takes that seat, it really does. And I'm okay with it now.

Back to our hawks, Hank and Mrs Hank. Soon, they found another tree on our farm to call home. They adapted quite easily and seemed to recognize that this journey, called life, is full of twists and turns. They've modeled for me that in life, we have to be willing to embrace change. Surrendering to this seemed easy for the hawks, not a sign of weakness, but a sign that a new adventure has begun. We'll likely see baby hawks next season, it's always a treat to see our family of hawks be a family and do hawk stuff. They endured a bend in the road, and they made the turn.

I hope it will be said of me one day, that though my tall trees came crashing down in mere seconds, I endured the bend in the road and made the turn.

David Advent

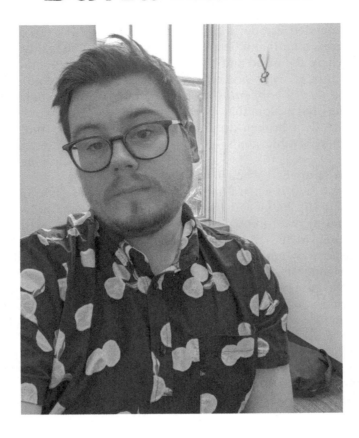

"I've experienced medical trauma after trauma due to RA, whether it's getting sick more often, or continuing to fight against internalized and externalized ableism. I am young, after all, and when most people think of a disability like RA, they don't think of a young man."

On a cold, gray morning in September I was laying in bed, trying to cover myself with the comforter, but was unable to use my hands and fingers. They felt like two large and rigid ice cubes. Sitting there with my paralyzed hands, I recalled the unusual pain and swelling that sporadically afflicted my joints over the previous year. Flares like this had happened with recurring frequency, but this was the worst one I had experienced. I was scared, confused, and unsure of what to do next to remedy the pain I was feeling.

With the encouragement of my friends and family, I finally contacted my primary care doctor, who, after reviewing the results of a laundry list of blood work, determined I needed to see a rheumatologist. A month later, the rheumatologist entered the room, examined my joints, and diagnosed me with severe rheumatoid arthritis (RA) and lupus. He immediately prescribed a detailed regimen of medications, to tamper the severity of the disease, including a biologic injectable drug that made me severely immunocompromised. The doctor left, and I sat alone.

I envisioned my life forming a glass orb which passed through my paralyzed hands and shattered onto the floor. I was in my senior year of college, at Florida State University, while working a part-time job, taking a full course load, completing an undergraduate honors thesis, and applying to graduate school. A debilitating chronic illness made achieving my goals much more difficult. But, I was determined to make the most of my college experience. I realized I had to make room for this illness to be part of my life, despite the incredible frustration I felt.

I drew inspiration on negotiating with my illnesses through a course I was taking on modern and contemporary poetry in my final semester. In this course, we completed a unit on the language poets and on the intersection between disability and poetics, discussing Susan Howe, Larry Eigner, and Jorie Graham. In this flurry of interdisciplinary and intermediality, both the disabled poets and the language poets experimented with new ways of writing poetry. Language poets engaged in visual art techniques, such as inverting words or forming them into specific shapes, to communicate their frustration with normative poetics. The disability poets I studied used these techniques to construct new ways of living outside of an ableist context. In these poets' experimentations, I saw my personal experience, with negotiating a chronic illness diagnosis represented, and this powerful representation charged me to advocate for inter- and trans-disciplinary approaches to life.

Despite the symptoms I was feeling, I began making peace with my chronic illnesses, and the results were empowering. I graduated on time from FSU with full honors, a 4.0 GPA, and a full-time job. I came to realize the strength, power, and agility I embodied. My life and career aspirations and my chronic illness, though seemingly contradictory, could exist together so long that I prioritized myself. I thereby found myself intersecting my personal experience, with a narrative of empowerment, self-actualization, and academic growth.

Obviously, RA has continued to be a part of my life even after college. I still continue taking humira and plaquenil to quell the raging storm of RA that infects my body. That's not to say that it always does the job. I've experienced medical trauma after trauma due to RA, whether it's getting sick more often or continuing to fight against internalized and externalized ableism. I am young, after all, and when most people think of a disability like RA, they don't think of a young man. Nevertheless, I have taken my experiences with RA into all aspects of my life, challenging myself to challenge this terrible disease, and make my experience known for everyone who has RA, so they don't feel alone like I did when I was first getting diagnosed.

Gittel Aguilar

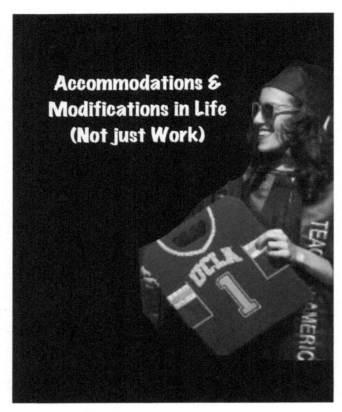

Accommodations & Modifications in Life (Not just Work)

"The accommodation felt like a privilege, and I definitely took advantage of it. I never thought of it as a necessity due to my limitations. It was simply part of my reality."

The earliest memory I have of chronic pain is from 2003. I was 15 years old, a sophomore in high school and an over-achieving student in my history class. That day we were watching a movie, and I was laying on the floor with my best friend. The teacher turned the lights on with the direction, "Okay, everyone head back to your seats." I promptly followed directions, but when I tried to stand up, something strange happened: I fell right back down.

"What are you doing?" my friend whispered.

"I don't know," I whispered back. *"I fell down,"* I added in a perplexed tone.

"I saw that," my friend said, amusement in her voice.

I tried to match it, but I remember feeling worried. It was the first time I was not in control of my body. If only I knew then what I know now. Countless tests, x-rays, and doctor visits later, I was still undiagnosed even though I knew something was wrong. The summer of my senior year in high school, I started conditioning with the cross country team, but I never made it to try outs. I would only last two weeks before the pain in my hip became so unbearable that I had to admit defeat. I thought it was because I went from not exercising at all to performing daily exercises. I blamed my efforts to be "healthy" and refused to exercise again. Let's be real, it was easier to adopt the identity of someone who hated exercising than to admit that I couldn't.

It really is a wonder that it took me so long to accept "disabled" as part of my identity, especially when I basically lived at the Office of Students with Disabilities all four years of college. It was through that office that I was able to get a specialized parking permit—the kind that professors have—so that I could drive to and from campus, instead of the usual 40 minute walk both ways. Sometimes I would even take naps in my car between classes. My favorite were the days when I would have the time in my schedule to drive back to the dining hall for lunch and not have to worry about packing or purchasing a meal.

"Hey, do y'all wanna head back up to the Hill with me for lunch?"

"Nah, don't feel like making the trek."

"I have my car! We ain't walking!"

"Oh hell yes!!"

I felt so popular because of my parking permit. It felt like a privilege, and I definitely took advantage of it; I never thought of it as a necessity due to my limitations. It was simply part of my reality. A seat cushion I won in a raffle at work also became part of my daily reality. It was one of those bleacher cushions fans use at football games with the school logo on it. It was my salvation! I took that thing everywhere, and I used it all the time! Sitting in class. Sitting at work. Undergrad graduation. Rides on the bus. Rides at Disneyland. Game days. Sitting at my favorite bar. Sitting at my new job. Grad school graduation.

If you knew me at this time in my life, you knew my seat cushion. I felt no shame using it, in fact, I got so many compliments for it, that I felt smart for doing so.

"*Oh, see? She brought her own cushion!*" someone would point it out to their friend.

"*Smaaaaaart,*" they'd respond, a trace of jealousy in their voices, as they sat on whatever hard surface was provided, while I sat comfortably on my cushion.

I'd smile and beam at how my alleviation was being applauded. Not once did I feel resentment at needing that accommodation. In fact, the more I practiced at shamelessly requesting accommodations and modifications for my jobs, the better I became. I followed the same pattern at all three of my places of employment. I'd have a good interview and at the end when they asked, *"What questions do you have for us?"* I'd make my case.

At my first job at the Customer Service department at the UCLA Store, I straight up said:

"*I see that the application says, 'I must be able to carry at least 40 pounds' or something like that, and I won't be able to do that.*"

"*Oh, don't worry about that!,*" was the reply.

At my second job as a teacher, I said, *"I understand that teachers have to give electives and the choices are between PE and art. Well, I'm unable to teach PE because of a hip problem I have—that's why the seat cushion—so I need to teach art."*

"*Sounds good! Writing that down in the notes now...*" and that's exactly what happened.

At my third job as a teacher at a different school, I said, *"I see that there's an Art teacher at this school, but no PE teacher. I won't be physically able to be a PE teacher–"*

"*Oh, you can modify the curriculum to fit your needs!*"

"*I'm glad, but that won't be enough for me. I'm afraid that if there's some sort of emergency, I will not be physically capable of helping the students, so I'm going to need someone else to take over my PE duties.*"

"*Totally doable! We'll get a T.A. to fill in for you, and you'll be there for supervisory reasons.*"

"*Perfect!*"

I never once felt ashamed for asking for these things. I knew that in order for me to get the job[s] done, these were the things I needed. It wasn't until I could no longer get the job done, that the shame started to set in. It was one thing to have undiagnosed chronic pain, but it was quite another to have multiple diagnoses of chronic illnesses that I would never "get well" from, not to mention having to acknowledge that I was unemployed due to disability due to these illnesses.

All of a sudden, the accommodations and modifications I asked for and needed seemed like asking for and needing "too much," like they added a ridiculous new level to the quality of my being "high maintenance," like they were yet another part of the burden I carried and that I was now projecting onto others, like they were yet another reason to choose not to be part of my life because it was too complicated.

How did I go from feeling so shameless when I was undiagnosed to having so much shame now that I am diagnosed?

I think internalized ableism and capitalism have a lot to do with it. Being unable to produce and contribute in the ways that society expects, and that I've grown to expect from myself, makes for quite a knock on one's self-esteem. It was different when the accommodations and modifications I was asking for were to help me produce and contribute as expected. But what about when I'm asking for accommodations and modifications simply because that is what I need to exist?

Where's the shame in that?

I'm proud of all I do to set myself up for success. I'm proud of all I do to advocate for myself and my needs. I'm proud of all I do to learn and relearn that my worth is not measured by my productivity. I'm proud of the progress I've made in feeling that vulnerability is far from a weakness, but one of my greatest strengths.

I have needs, and I refuse to be ashamed to get them met, regardless of diagnosis or expectations. When you're sick, the mentality switches. All of a sudden, basic survival is not only enough, it's full of things to celebrate—being able to sleep, being able to eat, being able full-stop, as well as having an appetite, having relief from pain, having a clear head, having energy. These are all things to celebrate and not take for granted because when you're sick, they're the first things to go. Being chronically ill means that I will be some level of sick forever, and there is no shame in using the tools I need to survive, in fact, it's something to celebrate!

Alexa Sutherland

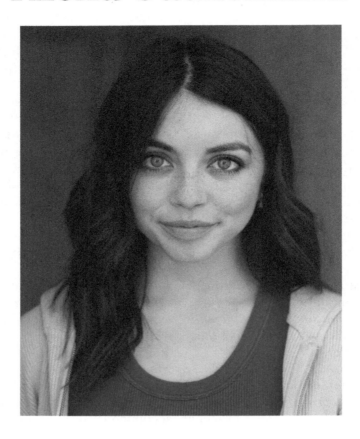

"In a roundabout way, I have my chronic illness to thank for leading me on a path that allowed me to further pursue my dreams in acting."

I'm a 24-year-old actress, writer, and advocate for individuals living with invisible disabilities. At just 15 months old, I was diagnosed with juvenile rheumatoid arthritis. From that point on I've tried just about every arthritis medication out there. Everything from pills, to injections, to IV infusions, along with pretty much every holistic measure under the sun. As a child, I was never able to play sports or involve myself in physical activities because it was too hard on my joints and caused too much pain. Instead, I loved performing, writing, and creating. I talked to just about anyone who would talk back to me, and admittedly loved being the center of attention.

For these reasons, my mom put me into the entertainment industry, when I was around three years old, where I grew up working on several print ads and commercials. As a kid, instead of getting dropped off at soccer practice after school, my mom drove me to auditions. Acting served as my "sport" in a sense. I met friends on the weekends in acting classes, or on set, and I absolutely loved it! It was where I was meant to be!

Fast forward to around the time I was entering high school where I was blessed to be in a medicated remission. I felt on top of the world and decided I was going to try out for the cheer team. A dream of mine that my family and I always thought was impossible due to my RA. But considering my health was at its highest, I wanted to give it a shot... and I made the team!! I was so elated, this was my first time being a part of a real "team". So when I started my freshman year in 2012, I stepped away from acting to focus on my studies...and cheerleading of course!

This all came to a crashing halt four months later when I experienced one of the biggest arthritis flares of my life. I was bedridden for weeks with swollen joints and immense pain. After being absent from school for nearly a month, my family and I made the decision to leave traditional high school, and re-enroll in an independent study once I got my health back on track. For the time being, I was completely reliant on my parents to help me with every small task. Life seemed impossible.

Weeks went on, and after starting a new medication and slowly getting my strength back, I started classes at the independent study program, which gave me the ability to work on schoolwork on my own terms, in the comfort of my own home. I ended up really thriving, in a work-at-your-own-pace environment, and graduated high school a year and a half early! With all that extra time on my hands and my health back in a steady place, I decided to get back into acting class and dedicated my time to working on my passion. This may sound crazy, but in a roundabout way, I have my chronic illness to thank for leading me on a path that allowed me to further pursue my interest in acting.

Since I decided to put my dreams first, I've had opportunities to work on several amazing projects! Some of my first television credits include MTV's 'Sweet Vicious', Disney Channel's 'Bizaardvark', and ABC's 'American Housewife' and 'Speechless'. My whole journey really came full circle this past year when I filmed my most recent project, 'Deadly Cheer Mom', which is now streaming for free on TUBI! It was such a fun experience filming a movie as a cheerleader, considering that's where this whole journey started for me!

When I say I have my disability to thank, I wholeheartedly believe that if I didn't suffer from that flare in my freshman year, I'd be a completely different person. I imagine I would've continued on with school, gone to college, joined a sorority, gotten a job in the field I was majoring in, and who knows where my stance with acting would be now!

I went to college online as well so I could keep my schedule open for acting opportunities. It was also beneficial knowing that online college would be easier for me and my health, as opposed to the traditional classroom setting. Sitting at hard desks, on someone else's timeline, didn't work for me since some days I'm pain-free, and other times it's hard to get up off the couch. School from home fits my lifestyle perfectly. I'm a firm believer that everything happens for a reason. I know I wouldn't be in the place I am today if my life path hadn't shifted.

I've had fears that one day I'll book a role that requires immense physical activity and my disability will limit me. However, I will just cross that bridge when I get there. And until then, all I can focus on is staying as healthy and happy as possible. My favorite quote is: "it's just a bad day, not a bad life." I try to remember this anytime I'm feeling down or am in pain. Everything will turn around, life will come full circle, and if it's meant to be...it will be! So thank you, chronic illness, for bringing me back to my roots so I could pursue this crazy dream of mine! I hope from here on out I can continue working on projects in the entertainment industry, and increase disability representation in film and television.

Aisling Maher

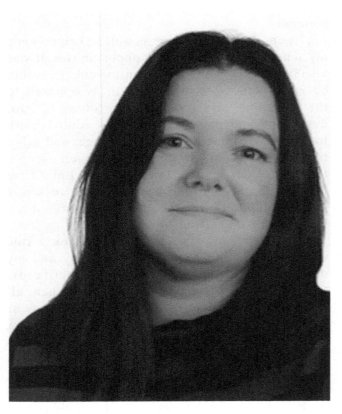

"I hand on heart believe that because I was in a high stress state for nearly three years, that when I started to relax and return to a "normal" pace of life, my body went into shock and decided enough was enough."

Before I was diagnosed, I was working in a very stressful, high-paced job that involved frequent international travel, multiple time zones, extremely long hours, and a large commute when I wasn't traveling.

I had two very young children, that I was trying to make sure were happy and healthy, and also a very understanding husband. I was frazzled, stressed, and felt incredibly guilty that I was away from home so much.

So, I did what I felt was the right thing and got a new job, working for a company that wasn't as stressful to work for and was more considerate of family life. I began to feel like myself again.

But then my body crashed. I couldn't function because of unrelenting fatigue, my hands and feet were swollen and painful and I just felt awful. Simple things like holding a steering wheel, wearing nice shoes, brushing or washing my hair, peeling vegetables, typing, and sometimes just sitting, standing, or lying in the same position for extended periods of time, caused me a lot of pain and discomfort. But, I still had to work and I still had to care for my family.

After a few months, I was diagnosed with rheumatoid arthritis. I started medication and it took a year and a half to find one that continues to work for me, and for this I am very grateful. I know that some people are not so lucky.

I hand on heart believe that because I was in a high stress state for nearly three years, that when I started to relax and return to a "normal" pace of life, my body went into shock and decided enough was enough.

I made a promise that I would never allow myself to get into a similar situation again. Your health is your wealth after all.

I had always been interested in using complementary therapies but when I was diagnosed I really took them seriously. BUT, I couldn't find anyone who specialized in inflammatory arthritis, or autoimmune conditions. So, I decided to learn how to do it myself and started to train as an aromatherapist, and from that many, many more therapies. Now, I help other women learn how to use complementary therapies as a support tool for rheumatoid arthritis.

I would never wish rheumatoid arthritis on anyone and would be very excited if a cure was found. But, I have to acknowledge that without it I wouldn't have my small business, or have met some wonderful people I now call friends. I'm grateful for that.

About the Creator

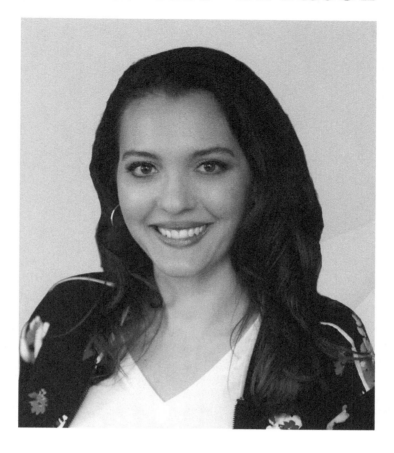

Effie Koliopoulos knew something was wrong when unrelenting fatigue led to joint pain, muscle aches, and random bruises on her body that disappeared just as quickly as they appeared. Over time she noticed that the same knuckles on each of her hands became slightly enlarged and inflamed, which would later occur in her right wrist, elbow, and knee. Her initial symptoms were brushed off as just 'growing pains' and nothing to worry about. After all, why should a young woman with a clean bill of health her whole childhood have any concerns? In 2004, those issues became validated with a diagnosis of juvenile idiopathic arthritis, formally known as juvenile rheumatoid arthritis. It wasn't until over a decade later, while recovering from a complex total knee replacement surgery at age 29, that the darkness of her difficulties began to slowly lose its power. The time of solitude began a journey of self-discovery, and purposeful action

and awakened a spark within to start sharing her story publicly and connect with people living with arthritis. After almost a year-long recovery, Effie launched her blog named Rising Above rheumatoid arthritis. This would be the beginning of many ideas to shine a light on life with arthritis, both independently and collectively. She was awarded the WEGO Health Rookie of the Year Award and is a recipient of the HealtheVoices Impact Fund which has helped fund her recent book project, Keeping It Real with Arthritis: Stories from Around the World. Her advocacy efforts can be found on AiArthritis, Creaky Joints, RheumatoidArthritis. net, NewLifeOutlook, Everyday Health, Healthline, and Good Housekeeping. Aside from everything arthritis and advocacy, she is a passionate storyteller at heart. Effie is currently working on other books and writing projects. She is a graduate of DePaul University and lives in Chicago.

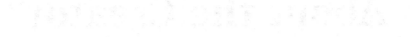

Made in the USA
Monee, IL
25 May 2023